The Naturopath In Your Hand

A Professional Protocol Book with Holistic Healing Protocols for Today's Most Common Health Issues

A PROFESSIONAL PROTOCOL BOOK BY

Diana M. Drake

Board Certified Traditional Naturopath

GOLDEN RAY
BOOK PUBLISHING

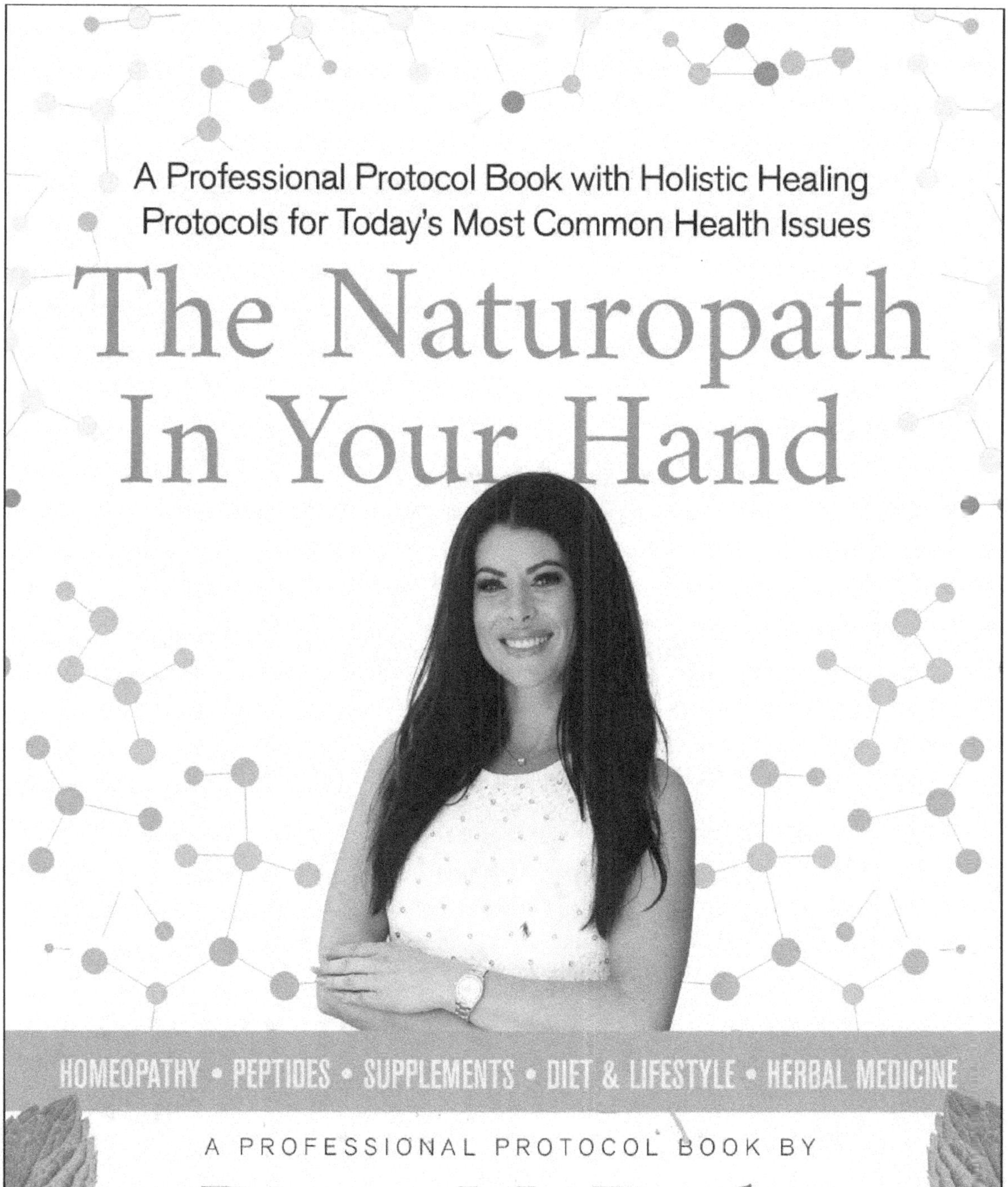
A Professional Protocol Book with Holistic Healing
Protocols for Today's Most Common Health Issues
The Naturopath
In Your Hand
HOMEOPATHY • PEPTIDES • SUPPLEMENTS • DIET & LIFESTYLE • HERBAL MEDICINE
A PROFESSIONAL PROTOCOL BOOK BY
Diana M. Drake
Board Certified Traditional Naturopath

The Naturopath In Your Hand

Homeopathy | Peptides | Supplements | Diet & Lifestyle | Herbal Medicine

Golden Ray Books is an imprint of Golden Ray Publishing, Inc.
7000 N. Central Expressway
Suite 501
Cheyenne, WY 82001
www.goldenraybooks.com

ISBN: 9798994508053

Editing, Copyediting, Proofreading, Text design and Composition,
Printed in the United States of America @2026
Distributed Digitally by Target, Walmart, Barnes & Noble Bookstores, Amazon, Kindle,
Indie Book Sellers.

Disclaimer: *The information provided in this book is for educational and informational purposes only. The content is not intended to be a substitute for professional medical advice, diagnosis, or treatment. Always seek the advice of your physician, mental health provider, or other qualified health provider with any questions you may have regarding a medical or health condition. Never disregard professional medical advice or delay in seeking it because of something you have read in this book.*

Contents

Diana M. Drake, BCTN · DMD Natural Medicine

Each chapter's protocols follow immediately after that chapter's discussion.
Use the Protocol Index on the next pages to jump straight to any protocol.

Protocol Index

All 44 protocols — each printed within its chapter

CHAPTER 1 · HORMONES & ANTI-AGING

CHAPTER 2 · WEIGHT, METABOLISM & CHOLESTEROL

CHAPTER 3 · STRESS & ENERGY

CHAPTER 4 · DIGESTIVE & GUT HEALING

CHAPTER 5 · DETOXIFICATION

CHAPTER 6 · IMMUNITY

CHAPTER 7 · PAIN

CHAPTER 8 · SKIN & HAIR HEALTH

CHAPTER 9 · SLEEP HEALTH

CHAPTER 10 · MENTAL WELLNESS

CHAPTER 11 · THYROID BALANCING

A NOTE FROM THE AUTHOR

A New Path to Healing

"You do not need to be afraid. It's time to learn, to understand, and to heal. It's time to break free."
- DIANA M. DRAKE

My personal story is a testament to the limitations of the Western medical business model, which often focuses on managing symptoms rather than addressing the root cause. It's a system that, for me, treated a number on a lab report but failed to recognize the deeper imbalances in my body. Now, as a Board-Certified Traditional Naturopath since 2018, my mission is to guide others toward their own "aha" moment and empower them to take control of their health. This journey of healing is not about fear; it's about education. Health is wealth and understanding how your body truly works is arguably the most important subject you will ever learn. Whether you are just beginning to question the traditional approach, are well into your wellness journey, or are a practitioner looking to build effective protocols, my new book is designed to support you.

Due to FDA regulations, my work—and this book—avoids common "disease names." Naturopaths do not treat diseases, as that term refers to the use of Western medical drugs, surgery, and vaccines. Instead, we focus on balancing groups of symptoms by working at the root cause. The book is broken down into the 10 most common categories of issues I've seen in my practice since 2018.

Inside, you will find "Protocol Sheets" clearly charted, "grab-and-go" documents that outline testing, product recommendations with dosing, and essential diet and lifestyle tips. These protocols are holistic, meaning they recognize that the body is a whole system that heals from the inside out. This means that the resolution of the symptom takes more time. Once your body's internal systems heal, the symptoms will resolve. While these protocols are based on the most common root causes, I want to emphasize that we are all bio-individuals. This book is not a substitute for a custom intake and evaluation with a naturopath, but it is the closest thing I could offer to get you started on the right path. I am thrilled to share this resource with you and help you navigate your healing journey. For those who need additional support beyond what this book offers, I am available for one on one and group consultations with both clients and practitioners. I also have memberships that allow access to natural healing at affordable prices

INTRODUCTION

Diana M. Drake, PhD.

Hello, practitioners, and those of you who are ready to take wellness into your own hands. It is wonderful to meet you here as you embark on this journey and act for your health. If you're reading this book, then you already know something is seriously wrong with the Western Medical system. Did you know that 23% of medical school funding comes from "Big Pharma"? Funding medical schools puts the pharmaceutical companies in a primary position to influence the education of our medical professionals. How can we have a medical system that puts the patient first when profits from selling drugs are such an influence? Medical schools teach how to diagnose and treat with pharmaceutical drugs and surgery. Meaning, if there is no drug under development by an Rx company, the treatment of specific symptoms and diseases may not make it into the medical curriculum. Additionally, we live in a "sick care" system, not a health care system, like we are led to believe. This sick care system is really a medical business model that profits in 3 distinct ways;

1. Hospital Stays: An average stay based on recent statistics:

The average length of an inpatient hospital stay in the United States is around 5.5 days. In a more recent figure daily costs average $24,680 for people with ample employer coverage. The number rises significantly if you receive surgery. A hospital is the only business where costs fluctuate, and pricing is not transparent. Hospitals can and will charge patients based on unclear processes that are not disclosed up front. What kind of business in America would you walk into, place an order, and only find out the total *after* you ask for the tab? To add insult to injury, "coverage" is based on how "good" an insurance policy you can afford or have. Leaving you to wonder - do those with better insurance get better care? Additionally, the total ticket price of your hospital bill, which you see, is sent to your insurance provider, where it is negotiated down, and only a portion is paid to the hospital. This vicious cycle of insurance "negotiating" causes providers to bill insurance companies an absolute premium in an attempt to get their maximum costs covered. For example, you may have a $120,000 hospital bill, which will be covered based on your insurance deductible and other factors. Still, the hospital may only receive $30k from your insurance provider for that bill. For the total billed amount, the percentage covered by insurance is usually much lower because the hospital's billed charges are not what the insurance company pays.

You can often get a better rate if you "cash pay" or "pay out of pocket" than you would get with insurance, because the hospital receives 100% of the money. Paying your bill may take some negotiating - especially after the case of an emergency, if life-saving care was already provided. The system, as it sits today, has many Americans opting out of the insurance system altogether and negotiating billing on their own.

2. Drugs & Required Vaccines:

America is the #1 consumer of prescription drugs in the entire world. Accounting for 50% of the worldwide sales revenue from Rx drugs. Yet Americans represent only 1/24th of the world's population, or 4% of humanity. America is also the sickest, most overweight country. I know there is a correlation here. The correlation is that American patients are led to believe that taking vaccines will *"prevent diseases"* and taking drugs will *"cure diseases."* The United States has THE MOST chronic diseases of any other country. The more we take, the more they make. The more we stay sick, the more "Big Pharma" profits from all of us. And they use the doctors to peddle their poison. Why on earth would any company make such a profitability change to their business model? The real problem with drugs and vaccines is that they do not address the root cause, which we will get into much more deeply later in the book.

3. Elective & Outpatient Surgeries:

According to HealthLeaders Media, surgical admissions (hospital stays involving surgery) accounted for 48% of hospital revenue and costs in one older study (2011), even though only ~29% of hospitalizations involved a surgical procedure. Elective inpatient and outpatient surgeries account for a significant share of hospital earnings. One study found that elective surgeries account for about 43% of gross hospital earnings in specific settings. It is in the hospital's best interests to recommend surgeries to patients, whether the patient needs them. In fact, there are many instances in which surgery can be avoided entirely when using a naturopathic protocol instead. Now I do not mean to say that surgery is "never" necessary. I am simply saying that if a business makes almost 50% of its revenue from surgery. You have a 50% chance of being recommended for surgery that you may OR may not need.

A couple of examples I would like to mention here - the first being Gallbladder removal surgery. Gallstones can often be cleared using a Gallbladder flush first to soften and eliminate the stones, thereby resolving any issues. Secondarily, neck, back, and shoulder surgery, depending on the case. With the incredible healing power of peptides, several studies have demonstrated that the body can reattach ligaments and muscles in animal models. It's been my personal experience from consulting with many chronic pain patients that back and neck surgery often does not get you better or help you move correctly.

"Sick Care" medicine has created a never-ending conveyor belt of "patients" who are purposely kept from understanding the true nature of healing. Instead, you are led to believe that taking vaccines and drugs will stop you from being sick. In doing this, you have lost our ability to know what keeps you healthy. Remember, your doctor has two jobs. First, diagnose the disease based on testing and/or symptoms, and second, treat the patient with drugs and/or surgery. Yes, there are some expansions on this, of course, but this is the primary focus of the Western medical business model.

Doctors have no training in nutrition, herbal medicine, or any preventive care except for disease screening, which is not prevention at all; it's simply *"early detection."* Proper education would involve the fundamentals of nutrition, detoxification, understanding of environmental toxic burden from food, water, air and soil, and the fundamental understanding of the body rather than a collection of individual parts. It can feel like the blind leading the blind. I challenge anyone to find a medical doctor who has this level of education working on a hospital floor or as a general practitioner. It doesn't exist. To get this kind of knowledge, a doctor must become disillusioned himself and go off the reservation to re-educate and re-structure their entire practice - which would be private and out of pocket but certainly not available to someone who walks in off the street for care at a hospital or medical office.

We deserve better. We deserve to be healthy and to know how our bodies work, how to nourish and protect ourselves. Do you want to break free from this cycle of *"sick care"*? Are you ready to listen to your intuition? We must listen to our inner voice that says, *"There must be a better answer out there."* Are you feeling SICK AND TIRED of asking your health care provider what is causing your *"dis-ease"* only to be ignored and/or told *"we're not sure"*? Are you tired of taking a recommended drug for your issue with no end in sight? Knowing that you are simply keeping the symptom in check, but have not created a healing space for your body? Enough is enough.

CHAPTER 1
Hormones & Anti-Aging

The absolute number one issue I have dealt with over the past several years in my practice is hormone imbalance in women. Hormone imbalances have a variety of root causes, but toxicity and blood sugar imbalance tend to be the most significant causes in cycling women. Menopause is, of course, the cause of many discomforts and drastic changes in a woman's body as she ceases to cycle. I had the absolute privilege of studying under Dr. Theresa Dale for several years before she passed away. She pioneered *"Homeopathic Hormone Rejuvenation"*, using homeopathic remedies to both balance and boost hormone levels - even in women who have had a full hysterectomy. In fact, you can also use homeopathy to balance hormones in people taking HRT (Hormone Replacement Therapy).

For those of you who are not experienced with homeopathy, homeopathic remedies are *"frequency"* remedies that have been prepared from original matter, then diluted and shaken again until the remedy has only the frequency imprint but almost no or negligible to none of the original ingredient(s). You can use anything from a poison - literally - to a vitamin, animal gland, or even an allergen to make a homeopathic remedy. A poison may be used as an antidote, just like snake venom is used as an antidote to a snake bite, or how a viral protein is used in a vaccine. Also, some herbs that are toxic at high doses have therapeutic use at smaller doses and are much safer taken homeopathically. To anyone nervous about taking a "toxic" herb, let me say this. ALL prescription drugs are toxic. Even an over-the-counter painkiller, for example, has therapeutic effects at a specific dose but can also kill you if you take too much.

The idea behind homeopathy is *"like cures like,"* so when you introduce the *frequency* of the poison into your body, you can read it differently, causing it to trigger detoxification of said poison. You may see a heavy metal detox remedy that contains the frequency of mercury or another metal. This list can be off-putting to someone reading the ingredients if they do not understand homeopathy. When you see an ingredient with a measurement behind it of 300 °C or 15X, for example, it refers to how much the original material has been diluted - also known as the "potency". A homeopathic tincture tastes like alcohol and water, which it primarily is.

When it comes to homeopathy and hormones, remedies can be stacked with several ingredients that include not only a single hormone, but many hormones of the endocrine system. The endocrine system is the body's network of glands and hormones that regulates growth, metabolism, reproduction, mood, and overall homeostasis. It includes glands such as the pituitary, thyroid, adrenals, pancreas, ovaries, and testes, which release hormones directly into the bloodstream. These hormones act as chemical messengers, traveling to target tissues to coordinate processes such as energy production, the stress response, sexual function, and tissue repair. Using homeopathy as a strategy, you can literally reboot your body's entire endocrine system rather than just focusing on one hormone that is out of balance. After all, your body relies on a complex cascade of *many* hormones coming from various glands in the body - and they are all connected.

One of the fallacies of Western medicine is to "add back" one or two of those low-level hormones through Hormone Replacement Therapy (HRT). While this can be an appropriate choice for many women in menopause, prescribing HRT or birth control to young, cycling women for anything other than contraception overlooks the root cause. This approach masks underlying imbalances rather than addressing them, often leading to deeper hormone issues, fertility challenges, and worsening symptoms once the medication is discontinued.

Contrary to what your doctor and the media may lead you to believe, your body can produce *all* the hormones it needs to survive from birth to death. Period. Yes, of course, there are exceptions for those born without a working pancreas or other parts of their endocrine system that didn't develop properly; however, I want you to understand that you can maintain proper hormone levels throughout your entire life. For example, did you know that once a woman's ovaries shut down after menopause, the adrenal glands continue to produce sex hormones? Sadly, none of our adrenal glands are healthy by this age due to the abuse of caffeine, alcohol, sugar, and the intense amount of stress from living in the modern world. Additionally, hormone health depends on a complex set of factors, including the air you breathe, the water you drink, your diet, exercise, the quality of your sleep, and your emotional health. Truly, hormone balance reflects health, not just your biological age.

The medical establishment fails to embrace the concept of your body as a natural, living system capable of self-repair. Instead, they want you to look *outside* of your body for a hormone product in the form of a one-size-fits-all solution. Whether we are talking about birth control pills or "Bio-Identical" hormones (shots, pills, pellets, patches, topical or vaginal creams), let's be very clear that these are all lab-made drugs that may have adverse side effects if not carefully monitored. Studies have shown that the use of HRT (Hormone Replacement Therapy) causes the body to shut down production of its own natural hormones and creates a dependency that can age every organ and bodily system. This may be ok for menopausal women and older men but is not ideal for a young person. I have also witnessed firsthand in hundreds of my own clients' hormone tests, that HRT can elevate - even skyrocket hormone levels to toxically high amounts. This overload taxes the adrenal glands, triggering the release of excessive cortisol, which worsens stress and fatigue. Additionally, many women report adverse side effects of these therapies, which is typically why they seek me out in the first place.

My goal here is for you to understand that you have natural, drug-free alternative options for your body. The key to natural medicine is first to ask yourself, *"Is this something my body can or should be doing on its own?"* before you agree to an endocrine-altering drug. Then, explore your options and familiarize yourself with various avenues before you decide. I would like to tell my clients this: *"Listen, the drug option will ALWAYS be there as a backup if all else fails. Let's look at drugs as the last stop rather than the first."* If you can adopt this principle, it will help guide your decisions for your health and well-being at all ages. Knowing this, I will run a naturopathic hormone & peptide protocol for 6 months on a young client first to see if we can get her endocrine system to respond. Only after exhausting that option will we look at HRT.

Please understand that I am not saying I am against HRT. In fact, there are many situations where that becomes the only option that will work, especially when it's age-related or if you have hormone-related fatigue, which will be covered later. What I am saying is that HRT needs to be properly monitored. It is important as a practitioner that I adapt to the changing times and new discoveries in this field. It is only recently (2025) that the FDA removed the black box cancer warning off HRT for women, especially those who have had a history of cancer. The caveat again - proper monitoring. It is very important to me that I offer *both* natural hormone rejuvenation, HRT and a hybrid of both depending on my client's needs. In 2026 DMD Natural Medicine proudly rolled out our telehealth platform giving access to telemedicine appointments in all 50 states allowing clients to virtually order labs and receive their customized hormone protocols from one of our 20 in network pharmacies for one convenient low monthly price. This platform is available to anyone by visiting our website and allows prescription peptides as well. Now let's jump in. I have created these checklists to help you understand if you potentially have a hormone issue that needs to be analyzed. Simply read each list and check off what applies to you.

Are you a teenage girl with any of the following symptoms related to your cycle? Check all the boxes below that may apply to you:

- ❑ Abnormal cycles or are "skipping" periods
- ❑ Painful cycles (above a 4 on a scale of 1-10)
- ❑ Heavy bleeding
- ❑ Breakouts/pimples on your face and body
- ❑ Severe negative symptoms around your cycle
- ❑ Confirmed cysts on your ovaries
- ❑ Dark facial hair
- ❑ Stubborn belly fat
- ❑ Craves sugar and carbs

If you checked 2 or more of the boxes above, I suggest you have an in-depth functional saliva hormone panel performed. The panel also checks your adrenal stress hormone (cortisol) 4 times throughout the day to properly evaluate your adrenal stress patterns. Additionally, the panel looks at excess androgens (androstenedione), an essential biomarker for potential Poly-cystic ovarian syndrome (PCOS) and menstrual irregularities. If you have been told you have PCOS by a medical doctor or if your doctor has ever said you have cysts on your ovaries, I strongly encourage you to read Dr. Casey Mean's *"Good Energy"* book to understand the relationship between metabolic health and your cycles. There is nothing more important than understanding what is happening in your own body.

It is now well understood that insulin resistance and poor blood sugar handling are the root causes of *most* PCOS cases and metabolic dysfunction. The pancreas helps to control blood sugar levels in your body. Blood sugar fluctuations can knock your sex hormones for a loop - these unbalanced hormones are what affect your cycles and the symptoms surrounding them, leaving you to assume you have *"menstrual issues"*. Meanwhile, the *real* root cause is pancreas and blood sugar issues. So again, if you treat these issues with birth control but do nothing to regulate your blood sugar, you are not healing anything. You would simply be putting on a band aid, that when removed, will still leave you to deal with the real issue. Take home here: get control of your blood sugar. Controlling your blood sugar is vital and is included in my hormone protocols when appropriate. If you are looking to conceive a child and you are having trouble doing so, or if you are getting pregnant but not able to carry to term, the same functional saliva test would be recommended for you. All my test recommendations and links will be available in the protocols listed at the end of each chapter and to make it easy you can find them.

Are you in perimenopause or are you going through menopause?
Check all the boxes below that may apply to you:

- ❑ Weight gain
- ❑ Stubborn belly fat
- ❑ Low sex drive / Lack of libido
- ❑ Brain Fog
- ❑ Poor skin elasticity / dry skin
- ❑ Hot flash & sweating
- ❑ Vaginal dryness
- ❑ Sleep Issues
- ❑ Mood Swings
- ❑ Adult acne

A saliva test offers crucial insights into adrenal health and cortisol patterns for women navigating this life change. Relying solely on Hormone Replacement Therapy (HRT) without addressing elevated cortisol—as revealed by the saliva test—creates a significant gap in proper treatment protocol; HRT alone doesn't resolve adrenal dysfunction. Furthermore, a single cortisol blood sample can be misleading. For instance, if you go to the doctor or lab for a 2 p.m. blood test that shows *normal* cortisol, it fails to detect potentially critical, dysfunctional diurnal patterns such as low cortisol in the morning and excessive levels at night. A dysfunctional diurnal pattern would, for example, explain waking incredibly tired and being wired at night. This missed nuance means a doctor completely overlooks essential information about your adrenal gland's health and function.

Are you a male of any age experiencing the following symptoms:
Check the boxes below that apply:

- ❑ Erectile dysfunction
- ❑ Low libido
- ❑ Low sperm count
- ❑ Hair loss
- ❑ Thinning hair
- ❑ Fatigue
- ❑ Stubborn belly fat
- ❑ Brain Fog
- ❑ Loss of muscle mass

As a naturopath who constantly recommends homeopathy, I want to mention that not everyone always responds to homeopathic medicine. It is essential to try the natural solutions first and to know that there is a backup net to catch you if all else fails. Homeopathy is great to balance the system and encourage native hormone production - it is also great to reduce menopause symptoms in women. But if you are looking to raise hormone levels significantly, then HRT (Hormone Replacement Therapy) may become a viable option for you. I see this especially apply to men with low testosterone. Should you need or choose to use HRT, there are some critical points I would like you to understand.

The first is: please monitor yourself often and use saliva testing at least once a year to compare to your blood results. I have seen hundreds of saliva hormone tests on women and men taking HRT that show testosterone, estrogens, and/or progesterone going way too high. When this happens, the hormone levels become toxic and dangerous. High levels of any of these hormones need to be avoided at all costs. Shockingly, many of my clients have reported to me that their hormone clinic physicians will only test their hormones every 2 years while using HRT. When using HRT, especially at the onset, more testing is not only necessary but required.

Our online telehealth platform includes the cost of follow up labs in your membership making it very easy to stay on track while checking your levels once you are taking HRT. Additionally, homeopathy can significantly help to harmonize HRT, making it much easier to balance and better for your body. I am providing a protocol for a combination of HRT and homeopathy for hormone "building". There are some excellent topical and oral HRT options available for DHEA, Estrogens and Progesterone. There are also good oral options for DHEA and Pregnenolone which are steroid precursor hormones meaning they turn into estrogens, testosterones and progesterone downstream. Again, do not use it without monitoring, and if you need testosterone, you will have to get it from our telehealth platform from a licensed medical provider, as it is a controlled substance.

Lastly, before we jump into the chapters, I want to note that most of my protocols call for iodine. From hormone balancing to energy, this vital element is essential, and most Americans are deficient in it. The deficiency is not from switching to sea salts or from not eating iodized table salt, but rather from exposure to too much toxic bromine. Bromine is a poisonous chemical to which we are constantly exposed to our food, homes, and the environment. Bromine is an active ingredient in fire-retardant chemicals, meaning it is sprayed on furniture such as couches, mattresses, curtains, and more. If you do not consciously choose to buy from stores that do not use fire-retardant sprays on their products, you are constantly being exposed to this chemical in your home. The problem is that this toxin kicks the iodine out of your hormone receptor sites - meaning a toxic chemical is plugging into a cellular receptor site where a hormone should be instead. Bromine falls into the category of "endocrine disruptors," and it doesn't stop there. All wheat and white flour in the United States contain bromine.

So, if you eat bread, pizza, bagels, pasta, crackers, and pastries made with non-organic flour, you are ingesting bromine. Golf courses also spray with chemicals that are heavy in bromine; this is why women who live on golf courses have a higher rate of breast cancer. The bromine accumulates in the glandular system, and the lack of iodine prevents the breast tissue from properly detoxifying. You may have heard that women who do not breastfeed have a higher chance of getting breast cancer. Breastfeeding is a detox pathway. Breastfeeding clears toxins that have built up in the breast tissue and surrounding lymphatics - unfortunately, by dumping the toxins into your baby's mouth - but it is a form of detoxification for the mother. The relationship between breast cancer and estrogen has more to do with xenoestrogens or estrogen-mimicking chemicals. A lot can be said about this, and there are many incredible books that you can read on this subject, such as *"Heal Breast Cancer Naturally"* by Dr. Veronique Desaulniers.

Before we dive into the protocols, we are going to start where all real healing begins — with your food. The Hormone Healing Diet is the foundation for every protocol in this book, and it is especially important for any hormone-balancing protocol. No supplement, peptide, or homeopathic remedy can fully do its job while your body is still being fed the very things that threw your hormones off in the first place. So let's start here, together — follow the diet on the pages that follow as closely as you can, and give your body what it needs to come back into balance.

DIETARY PROTOCOL

The Hormone Healing Diet

ⓧ ELIMINATE ⓛ REPLACE WITH ⊕ INCREASE ⊝ MODERATE

ⓧ ELIMINATE — ALL STIMULANTS

REMOVE

Caffeine | Coffee | Green, white & black tea | Chocolate | Sugar | Candy | Soda | Corn syrup | Baked goods | Canned / bottled fruit juices | Salad dressings with added sugar

REPLACE WITH

- **Coffee alternatives:** www.Teeccino.com
- **Dandelion coffee:** www.DandyBlend.com
- **Organic herbal tea:** lemon, ginger, jasmine, herbal blends, chamomile, citrus, etc.
- **Kombucha** in *small* amounts (contains both sugar and caffeine) — 1 shot per day, or several days weekly, is the limit if you must have it. www.TheFermentingFairy.com

ⓧ ELIMINATE — PROCESSED GRAINS

REMOVE

Wheat / gluten bread | Pasta | Pizza | Bagels | Baked goods | Crackers

REPLACE WITH

- **Crackers:** seed crackers
- **Bread:** sprouted grains, almond flour
- If you do have bread on occasion, please use **organic** wheat flour in sourdough.
- Learn to bake with nut flours and natural sugars like honey, monkfruit, maple syrup or agave.
- **Pizza crust:** cauliflower crust (make sure it is free of seed oils / canola oil).
- For **crunchy snacks**, have fresh veggies with hummus or other dips.
- **Potato chips** with no pesticides, made with beef tallow: www.vandycrisps.com

ELIMINATE — SEED OILS

REMOVE

- Canola (even "organic, cold-pressed")
- Sunflower oil & lecithin
- Soy oil & lecithin
- Rapeseed oil
- Grapeseed oil
- Olive oil "blends" (use pure only)
- Commercial / restaurant dressings
- Mayonnaise (contains canola)

REPLACE WITH

For cooking:

Organic grass-fed butter, coconut oil, avocado oil, and beef tallow (they have a higher smoke point).

For dressings:

Cold-pressed, organic olive oil — the greener the better. Should come in dark glass; avoid plastic and tins.

If you need to fry something, use **beef tallow**.

MEDICINAL SEED OILS — BENEFICIAL IN THE RIGHT FORM

Black cumin — supports immunity & inflammation

Flaxseed — omega-3 rich; supports hormone & heart health

Pumpkin seed — rich in zinc & phytosterols

Hemp seed — proper omega balance

Rosehip — rich in vitamin A & antioxidants

Evening primrose — rich in gamma-linolenic acid (GLA)

Sea buckthorn — contains omega-7s

Pomegranate seed — antioxidant & hormone balancing

Sesame seed — rich antioxidant

Grape seed — antioxidant, rich in proanthocyanidins

ELIMINATE — DEEP-FRIED FOODS

REMOVE

- Potato chips
- French fries
- Fried chicken
- Breaded tenders & nuggets
- Donuts
- Egg rolls
- Tempura
- Calamari
- Fried fish / fish sticks
- Mozzarella sticks

REPLACE WITH

- Baked or pan-fried items instead, cooked with the proper oil or fat.
- Use gluten-free or non-GMO corn-based breading if "breading" something to fry.
- If you have to have something fried, make sure it's cooked in **beef tallow**.

⊕ INCREASE — ORGANIC GREENS

Spinach · Romaine · Green & red leaf lettuce · Butterhead lettuce · Arugula · Watercress · Endive · Escarole · Kale · Swiss chard · Collard greens · Mustard greens · Beet greens · Turnip greens · Dandelion greens · Cabbage · Brussels sprouts · Micro-greens

> **How to get them in:** Raw salads are a great way to get greens in. Cold-pressed fresh juice from a slow masticating juicer is an especially good way to work in greens or herbs you don't like to eat whole.

⊕ INCREASE — WILD-CRAFTED FRESH HERBS

Basil — salads, pesto, tomato dishes, pasta, eggs

Oregano — Italian & Greek dishes, roasted veggies, meats

Thyme — roasted meats, potatoes, soups, stews

Rosemary — strong, piney; roasted meats, bread, potatoes

Sage — earthy; poultry, beans, butter sauces

Parsley — garnish, tabbouleh, sauces, soups

Chives — delicate onion; potatoes, eggs, salads

Dill — pickles, fish, potatoes, yogurt sauces

Chervil — delicate anise; eggs, salads, fish

Sorrel — tangy; soups, salads, sauces

Nasturtium — peppery leaves & flowers; salads, garnishes

Fennel fronds — salads, fish, soups

Bay leaves (fresh) — soups, stews, braises (remove before serving)

Tarragon — subtle licorice; chicken, fish, cream sauces

Marjoram — mild oregano-like; soups, roasted meats

Cilantro — tacos, curries, salsas, soups

Mint — salads, spring rolls, teas, lamb, yogurt sauces

Thai basil — spicy-sweet; stir-fries, curries, pho

Lemongrass — soups, curries, teas

Shiso (perilla) — Japanese dishes, sushi, salads, wraps

Curry leaves — Indian curries, lentils, soups

Za'atar herbs — thyme, oregano, marjoram, sumac; flatbreads, dips

Fenugreek leaves (methi) — curries, breads, bean dishes

Lovage — celery-like; soups, broths, stews

Culantro — stronger than cilantro; soups, stews, sofrito

Epazote — traditional in beans & Mexican cooking

Cuban oregano — bold; marinades, meats, stews

⊕ INCREASE — ORGANIC VEGGIES

CRUCIFEROUS

Broccoli · Cauliflower · Brussels sprouts · Cabbage (green, red, napa, savoy) · Bok choy · Kohlrabi · Radishes

ROOT VEGETABLES

Carrots · Beets · Turnips · Parsnips · Rutabaga · Sweet potatoes · Yams · Daikon · Burdock root

ALLIUM FAMILY

Garlic · Onions (yellow, red, white, shallots) · Leeks · Scallions · Chives

NIGHTSHADES

Tomatoes · Eggplant · Bell peppers · Chili peppers · Potatoes

OTHER VEGETABLES & PODS

Corn · Green beans · Snow peas · Sugar snap peas · Okra

MUSHROOMS

White button · Cremini · Portobello · Shiitake · Maitake · Oyster · Enoki

GOURDS & SQUASH

Cucumbers · Zucchini · Yellow squash · Pumpkin · Spaghetti squash · Butternut squash · Acorn squash

⊕ INCREASE — FRUITS

POME FRUITS

Apples · Pears (Bartlett, Anjou, Bosc, Asian) · Quince

CITRUS

Oranges · Grapefruit · Lemons · Limes · Tangerines · Pomelo

STONE FRUITS

Peaches · Plums · Nectarines · Apricots · Cherries · Mangoes

BERRIES

Strawberries · Blueberries · Blackberries · Raspberries · Cranberries · Gooseberries · Currants · Mulberries

TROPICAL

Bananas · Pineapple · Papaya · Guava · Lychee · Passion fruit · Dragon fruit · Rambutan

MELONS

Watermelon · Cantaloupe · Honeydew · Galia · Canary

GRAPES & VINE FRUITS

Red grapes · Green grapes · Concord grapes · Kiwi (green & golden)

EXOTIC / SPECIALTY

Pomegranate · Figs · Dates (Medjool, Deglet Noor) · Persimmon · Starfruit · Sapote · Jackfruit

⊕ INCREASE — BEANS & LEGUMES

COMMON BEANS

Black beans · Pinto beans · Kidney beans (red & white) · Navy beans · Great Northern · Cannellini · Adzuki

LENTILS

Green · Brown · Red (split) · Yellow · Black (Beluga) · French (Puy)

CHICKPEAS & PEAS

Chickpeas (garbanzo) · Green peas · Split peas (yellow, green) · Black-eyed peas

SOY-BASED

Edamame · Soybeans (dried) · Mung beans · Tempeh (fermented) · Natto (fermented)

SPECIALTY & LESSER-KNOWN

Fava (broad) beans · Lupini beans · Winged beans · Pigeon peas (toor dal) · Hyacinth beans

⊕ INCREASE — NUTS & SEEDS

TREE NUTS

Almonds · Walnuts · Pecans · Hazelnuts · Brazil nuts · Cashews · Pistachios · Macadamia

OTHER NUTS & NUT-LIKE

Peanuts (legume) · Pine nuts · Chestnuts

NUTRIENT-DENSE SEEDS

Chia — omega-3s, fiber, protein; gels when soaked

Flax (ground) — omega-3s & lignans; hormone support

Hemp hearts — protein; balanced omega-3:6 ratio

Pumpkin (pepitas) — zinc, magnesium, iron

Sunflower — vitamin E, selenium, healthy fats

Sesame — calcium, copper, lignans; also tahini

SPECIALTY / LESSER-KNOWN SEEDS

Poppy — baking; calcium & manganese

Nigella (kalonji) — antioxidant & anti-inflammatory

Mustard — supports digestion & circulation

Coriander — aromatic; aids digestion

Fennel — soothes digestion, freshens breath

Cumin — digestion, blood-sugar balance

Fenugreek — bitter-sweet; curries & remedies

Cardamom — antioxidant & digestive

> **Tips for using seeds:** Eat them raw, roasted, or ground into smoothies, salads, yogurt, baked goods, or dressings. Store in airtight containers in the fridge or freezer to keep the oils from going rancid. Grind flax before eating for maximum absorption (whole flax passes through undigested). Mix different seeds ("seed cycling") for variety in nutrients.

⊕ PLANT-BASED PROTEIN SOURCES

PER CUP COOKED, UNLESS NOTED

Lentils	18 g	Quinoa	8 g · complete
Edamame	17 g	Farro	7 g
Split peas	16 g	Peanuts	7 g / oz · legume
Chickpeas / garbanzo	15 g	Buckwheat	6 g · gluten-free
Black beans	15 g	Oats	6 g
Kidney beans	15 g	Sunflower seeds	6 g / ¼ cup
Pinto beans	15 g	Almonds	6 g / oz (~23)
Teff	10 g	Pistachios	6 g / oz
Hemp seeds	10 g / 3 tbsp · complete	Brown rice	5 g
Amaranth	9 g · complete	Chia seeds	5 g / 2 tbsp
Pumpkin seeds / pepitas	9 g / ¼ cup	Flax seeds (ground)	4 g / 2 tbsp

MODERATE — ANIMAL PRODUCTS

≤ 30% OF DIET · MUST BE ORGANIC

RED MEATS

Beef (steak, ground, roasts) · Lamb · Venison · Bison / buffalo · Goat

POULTRY

Chicken · Turkey · Duck · Goose · Quail

FISH & SEAFOOD

Salmon · Sardines · Mackerel · Herring · Anchovies · Tuna · Trout · Cod · Halibut · Snapper · Shrimp, crab, lobster · Clams, mussels, oysters, scallops · Squid · Octopus

EGGS

Chicken eggs · Duck eggs · Quail eggs

DAIRY

Milk (cow, goat, sheep) · Yogurt / Greek / kefir · Cheese (cheddar, mozzarella, feta, parmesan, goat) · Cottage cheese · Cream / heavy cream · Butter / ghee

OTHER ANIMAL PRODUCTS

Organ meats (liver, heart, kidney, tongue) · Bone broth · Gelatin / collagen

CLINICAL PROTOCOL

Menopause Protocol – 100% Natural

BY **DIANA M. DRAKE, BCTN** · DMD NATURAL MEDICINE

① RECOMMENDED LABS

Access Medical Labs — OpenDx Saliva Hormone Supreme

Test initially to evaluate hormones and adrenal health. Hormones will be lower — that is normal. Ideally, aim to get them into range for the season of your cycle. If you cannot get hormone function up, that is okay — use the protocol to help with the negative symptoms associated with this life change. If adrenal cortisol is off, use the recommendations below to help balance.

② RECOMMENDED PRODUCTS

CORE PROTOCOL

DR. DALE'S

MenoGel

DOSE 1–2 pumps in the AM & PM on the inner arm, Monday–Friday only.

Start with 1 pump and work your way up. Once symptoms abate, you need to **lower** the dose — this is important to keep symptoms from returning. Do not use caffeine, even on days off. If this remedy isn't working for you, you may not have properly removed all stimulants from your diet and may not be fully following the hormone diet.

DR. DALE'S

Berberine Pro

DOSE 1–2 caps with every meal.

Supports proper blood sugar balance and may help balance post-meal sugar spikes. If you have stubborn belly fat or weight gain, Berberine Pro is required. If you do not struggle with belly fat or weight gain, you do not need to take it.

DR. DALE'S

Full Body Detoxification Kit

DOSE Liver Pro, Kidney Pro & Whole Body Immune Pro: 3 caps of each, three times daily with meals. Colon Pro: 1–2 caps with meals. *Reduce if diarrhea occurs.*

Run every spring and fall for 30 days, and at the onset of beginning MenoGel. If you have never done a detox before, or if you still have symptoms after 30 days, you may need to run this program several times. Take a 1–2 week break between cycles.

DR. DALE'S

Optimal Multi-Pro

DOSE 1–2 capsules daily with the first meal of the day.

Contains foundational nutrition and adrenal support with adaptogenic herbs for overall nutrition and adrenal support.

DR. DALE'S

Adaptogen Pro

DOSE 1–2 caps with the first 2 meals of the day.

A great add-on if severe adrenal imbalance is present — if you are tired, stressed out, and sensitive to stress. Taken earlier in the day it will help with energy; taken closer to the evening it will help support sleep. *Not necessary if adrenal cortisol is in balance and you live a low-stress life.*

DR. DALE'S

Vitamin D & K

DOSE 1 capsule daily with a meal. May increase to 2 caps daily in winter, especially in a cold climate.

Vitamin D is an important precursor to hormone production, as well as bone and immune support as you age. This formula is blended with Vitamin K for best absorption.

DR. DALE'S

Nano-Ionic Iodine

DOSE 30 drops daily with water.

Iodine is imperative for every woman for hormone, thyroid, and breast health. If you are iodine deficient, you may want to start with the Bio-Iodine cap, as it is more potent.

DR. DALE'S

Nano-Ionic Multi-Mineral with Silica

DOSE 30 drops daily in water.

Supports proper mineralization, especially when drinking filtered water.

BIOTICS RESEARCH

FeZyme Iron Supplement

DOSE 1 tablet daily.

Iron is important, especially if you know that you run low. If you have never been told you are low on iron, this may not be necessary — especially once you are done cycling.

NATURA HEALTH

Meno-Breeze

DOSE 3 capsules daily.

Botanical support formulated to ease menopausal transition symptoms.

③ RECOMMENDED PEPTIDES

REJUVATIDE PEPTIDES · GLP-1 FAMILY

Metabolic Peptide (Sema, Reta, Tirz, Maz)

DOSE Reconstitute a 10 mg bottle with 1 mL bacteriostatic water. Dose 10–25 units once weekly on the same day, *or* once every 5 days. Start low and increase by 5 units per week until the "food chatter" lessens. Cycle 12 weeks on, 4 weeks off.

Fast weight loss and having no appetite is **not** the goal — be gentle and go slow while the peptide works on cellular metabolism. On your 4 weeks off, juice cleansing, water fasting, and a calorie-restricted diet help keep the weight down; you can also cycle onto a different peptide, such as AOD (which works on a different pathway) during the rest cycle. All GLP peptides — regardless of their common reference of being a 1, 2, or 3 — are technically GLP-1; they may work on one or more pathways. Try different formulas to see which one works best for you. Supports weight loss, food cravings, and blood sugar balance. Best injected into sub-Q fat on the abdomen, thigh, or back of the arm.

REJUVATIDE PEPTIDES · GROWTH-HORMONE SECRETAGOGUE BLEND

CJC-1295 5 mg + Ipamorelin 5 mg (or Tesamorelin 10 mg, or Sermorelin 10 mg)

DOSE Reconstitute a 10 mg bottle with 2 mL bacteriostatic water. Dose 10–25 units. Cycle 8 weeks on, 2–4 weeks off. Use 5 days on, 2 days off.

A 10 mg blend to support lean muscle mass in aging women. For fat burning, inject before a fasted cardio workout. For muscle building, take after a workout, then fast for 90 minutes. On a non-workout day, or if not working out, take before bed.

REJUVATIDE PEPTIDES

PT-141 10 mg

DOSE Mix with 2 mL bacteriostatic water. Begin at 10 units for both males and females, AM or PM as needed.

For low libido and sexual desire.

⚠ DO NOT USE WITH UNMANAGED HIGH BLOOD PRESSURE

④ RECOMMENDED PRODUCTS — LOCAL SUPPORT

BEZWECKEN

Hydration Ovals

> DOSE Insert one vaginally once daily, or every few days, for vaginal dryness associated with menopause.

Choose the hormone-free formula, or a formula with hormones that delivers local hormones and moisture to the vaginal tissue when inserted.

⑤ ADDITIONAL PROTOCOL NOTES

1. **Stop the use of stimulants.**
2. **Caffeine must be 100% avoided** on this protocol, or it will stop the homeopathy from working. Please wean yourself off by 25% less every week. Coffee substitutes can be found at www.Teeccino.com.
3. **Mint** — such as in tea and essential oils on the skin — should be used in moderation, as mint may interfere with homeopathic remedies.
4. **Sugar is also a stimulant** and should be avoided.

CLINICAL PROTOCOL · 100% NATURAL

Abnormal Cycles, Ovarian Cysts & Hormonal Skin Breakouts

BY **DIANA M. DRAKE, BCTN** · DMD NATURAL MEDICINE

① RECOMMENDED LABS

ACCESS MEDICAL LABS

OpenDx Saliva Hormone Supreme

TIMING Test initially, then every 2 months as follow-up.

The key you are looking for is elevated **Androstenedione**, an indicator of excess androgens. Out-of-range cortisol levels matter as well — the combination may signal poor blood sugar handling, a root cause of your symptoms.

ZRT LABORATORY

Cardio-Metabolic Panel

A comprehensive panel to assess potential metabolic dysfunction, which is often a root cause of these issues. **If imbalances are present, blood sugar balancing is imperative** — take processed sugar and processed grains out of the diet.

VARIOUS OPTIONS AVAILABLE

Food Sensitivity Test

Recommended if acne and breakouts are present. Choose from the available testing options.

US BIOTEK

GI Microbiome Test — GI-Basic Profile

Assesses the gut microbiome, which frequently contributes to hormonal and skin symptoms.

② THE HORMONE KIT

HOMEOPATHIC · USE PER LAB RESULTS

DR. DALE'S NUFEM #1

Homeopathic Progesterone Topical Spray (IF PROGESTERONE IS LOW)

DOSE 1–4 sprays on the inner arm, Days 12–28 of your cycle. 5 days on, 2 days off.

Use if progesterone is low or needs balancing. Run this protocol for 6 months. If progesterone doesn't come up on follow-up testing and periods do not start to normalize, a topical bio-identical progesterone may be necessary to raise levels — continue this homeopathic formula alongside the HRT to help harmonize the protocol.

If progesterone is **high**, use the Original Hormone-Free formulas instead.

DR. DALE'S NUFEM #2

Homeopathic Estrogen Topical Spray (IF ESTROGEN IS LOW)

DOSE 1–2 sprays, Days 1–28 of your cycle. 5 days on, 2 days off.

Use if estrogen(s) are low. Continue to monitor estrogen levels via saliva testing. You may keep using this in combination with non-homeopathic formulas if you end up needing HRT; a topical bio-identical estrogen may be required if estrogens continue to be too low to normalize the cycle. Monitor carefully if bringing in HRT.

If estrogen is **high**, use the Original Hormone-Free formulas instead.

DR. DALE'S NUFEM #3

Homeopathic Testosterone Spray (IF TESTOSTERONE IS LOW)

DOSE 1–4 sprays on the inner arm, Days 12–28 of your cycle. 5 days on, 2 days off.

Use if testosterone is low.

If testosterone is **high**, use the Original Hormone-Free formulas instead.

DR. DALE'S

Bio Age Reverse Drops

DOSE 5 drops under the tongue, AM & PM, Monday–Friday.

Supports overall hormone balance across the endocrine system and completes the hormone kit.

DR. DALE'S

MBM/NER Female #13

Supports overall hormone balance for the female endocrine system specifically, and completes the hormone kit.

③ SKIN & ANDROGEN SUPPORT

SKIN NATUROPATHIC

Hormonal Breakouts

DOSE 2–5 capsules, 3 times daily with meals. Find the dose you respond to — start low and work your way up.

Useful in this scenario even if breakouts are not present. This herbal formula supports the balance of excess androgens and blood sugar and encourages a healthy ovulation cycle. It contains most of the recommended ingredients for women with PCOS in one convenient supplement.

If you are not taking the full 5 caps × 3 daily, add **Dr. Dale's NAC Pro** to reach a full 1500 mg per day. See the separate NAC instructions.

SKIN NATUROPATHIC

Derma-Detox

> **DOSE** 2–4 caps with meals, to bowel tolerance. Reduce dose if diarrhea occurs.

Detoxification should continue until symptoms are reduced by 80% — this may take over 6 months. Finish a bottle, take a 2-week break, then repeat.

④ FOUNDATIONAL SUPPORT

DR. DALE'S

Vitamin D & K

> **DOSE** 1 capsule daily with food. Up to 2 daily in winter, especially in a cold climate.

Vitamin D is an important precursor to hormone health; this blend with Vitamin K supports proper absorption and bone health.

DR. DALE'S

Nano-Ionic Iodine

> **DOSE** 20+ drops daily with water.

Iodine is critical for every hormone protocol — it is needed to feed and detox the glandular system and tissues.

BIOTICS RESEARCH

FeZyme

> **DOSE** 1 tablet daily in the AM.

Iron is important, especially if you know you run low. Women lose more iron than men due to menstruation, so it is important to replenish. The only reason you would not need an iron supplement is if a test shows your levels are too high.

⑤ RECOMMENDED PEPTIDES

REJUVATIDE PEPTIDES · GLP-1 FAMILY

GLP-1 Metabolic Peptide — single, dual or triple agonist, 10 mg

> **DOSE** Reconstitute with 1 mL bacteriostatic water. Inject 2.5–10 units once weekly on the same day, into sub-Q fat. Start low and work your way up if needed.

This should help manage cycles, inflammation, and fertility — it is not used, in this case, as an appetite suppressant.

This protocol is provided for educational purposes and is intended for patients under the care of a qualified practitioner. It is not a substitute for individualized medical advice, diagnosis, or treatment. Hormone and homeopathic recommendations should be guided by saliva hormone testing and ongoing monitoring. Do not begin, stop, or adjust any hormone, peptide, or supplement without consulting your provider — particularly if you are pregnant or nursing, taking medications, or managing a medical condition.

CLINICAL PROTOCOL · 100% NATURAL

Painful & Heavy Cycles

Excess androgens & potential ovarian cysts. If hormonal acne is present, see the Hormonal Breakout Protocol.

BY **DIANA M. DRAKE, BCTN** · DMD NATURAL MEDICINE

① RECOMMENDED LABS

ACCESS MEDICAL LABS

OpenDx Saliva Hormone Supreme

ZRT LABORATORY

Cardiometabolic Profile

TESTING FREQUENCY & WHAT TO LOOK FOR

Test initially and every 2 months as follow-up. The key you are looking for is elevated **Androstenedione**, an indicator of excess androgens. Out-of-range cortisol levels matter as well — the combination may be a sign of poor blood sugar handling, and a root cause of your symptoms. If **A1C is above 5.2**, blood sugar imbalance may be a root cause of your issues.

⚠ **Elevated 17-OHP → see an endocrinologist.**
Elevated 17-OHP — especially alongside cortisol imbalance and elevated androgens — may point to an **adrenal** root cause rather than ovarian or blood sugar. This protocol may still support balance and help with symptoms, but please have an endocrinologist review any out-of-range 17-OHP for a proper diagnosis.

② THE HORMONE KIT

HOMEOPATHIC · USE PER LAB RESULTS

DR. DALE'S NUFEM #1

Homeopathic Progesterone Topical Spray (IF PROGESTERONE IS LOW)

DOSE 1–4 sprays on the inner arm, Days 12–28 of your cycle. 5 days on, 2 days off.

Use if progesterone is low or needs balancing. If, after 6 months of homeopathy, progesterone is not coming up in labs, it may be necessary to bring in topical bio-identical progesterone — this must be carefully monitored. Continue the homeopathy alongside the HRT, as it will help harmonize the protocol.

If progesterone is **high**, use the Original Hormone-Free Progest formula instead.

DR. DALE'S NUFEM #2

Homeopathic Estrogen Topical Spray (IF ESTROGEN IS LOW)

DOSE 1–2 sprays, Days 1–28 of your cycle. 5 days on, 2 days off.

Use if estrogen(s) are low. Even if estrogens are low, if progesterone is lower this may still be an **"estrogen dominant"** profile — progesterone will need to come up and be properly balanced in ratio with estrogens. Estrogens may require HRT if homeopathy alone cannot raise production within 6 months.

> If estrogen is **high**, use the Original Hormone-Free formula instead.

③ EXCESS ANDROGEN SUPPORT

SKIN NATUROPATHICS

Hormonal Breakouts Female

DOSE Capsules 3 times daily with meals. Find the dose you respond to — start low and work your way up.

An all-in-one formula designed to balance blood sugar and excess androgens that cause negative hormonal symptoms in women.

DR. DALE'S · FULL-BODY DETOX

Liver Pro, Colon Pro, Kidney Pro & Whole-Body Immune Pro

DOSE 3 caps of each with each meal (2–3 times daily, depending on how many meals you eat), 5 days on, 2 days off. Colon Pro: 1–2 capsules with each meal — reduce by 1 if diarrhea occurs.

Continue detoxification month by month until your periods are lighter and pain is down to 3 or less out of 10. Detox, then rest for 2 weeks, and repeat.

④ FOUNDATIONAL SUPPORT

DR. DALE'S

Nano-Ionic Iodine

DOSE 20+ drops daily with water.

Iodine is critical for every hormone protocol — it is needed to feed and detox the glandular system and tissues.

BIOTICS RESEARCH

FeZyme

DOSE 1 tablet in the AM.

Iron is important, especially if you know you run low. Women lose more iron than men due to menstruation, so it is important to replenish. The only reason you would not need an iron supplement is if a test shows your levels are too high.

DR. DALE'S

Vitamin D & K

> DOSE 1 capsule daily with food. Up to 2 daily in winter, especially in a cold climate.

An important precursor to hormone health; this blend with Vitamin K supports proper absorption and bone health.

SKIN NATUROPATHICS

Lighter Cycles

> DOSE 3 capsules, 3 times daily, ongoing.

Supports lighter, less painful cycles.

⑤ RECOMMENDED PEPTIDES

REJUVATIDE PEPTIDES · GLP-1 FAMILY

Metabolic Peptide (Sema, Tirz, Reta, Maz) — single, dual or triple agonist, 10 mg

> DOSE Reconstitute the 10 mg bottle with 1 mL bacteriostatic water. Inject 3–5 units weekly on the same day, or every 5 days.

Studied for its ability to balance blood sugar and insulin pathways — often a root cause associated with these issues.

⑥ PROTOCOL NOTES

STOP ALL STIMULANTS

1. **Caffeine must be 100% avoided** on this protocol, or it will stop the homeopathy from working. Please wean yourself off by 25% less every week. Coffee substitutes can be found at www.Teeccino.com.
2. **Mint** — such as in tea and essential oils on the skin — should be used in moderation, as mint may interfere with homeopathic remedies.
3. **Sugar is also a stimulant** and should be avoided.

This protocol is provided for educational purposes and is intended for patients under the care of a qualified practitioner. It is not a substitute for individualized medical advice, diagnosis, or treatment. Hormone and homeopathic recommendations should be guided by saliva hormone testing and ongoing monitoring. Any out-of-range 17-OHP should be evaluated by an endocrinologist. Do not begin, stop, or adjust any hormone, peptide, or supplement without consulting your provider — particularly if you are pregnant or nursing, taking medications, or managing a medical condition.

CLINICAL PROTOCOL · 100% NATURAL

Female Fertility Support

Fertility issues · cannot conceive · cannot carry to term

BY **DIANA M. DRAKE, BCTN** · DMD NATURAL MEDICINE

> It is imperative for fertility that you have healthy ranges of sex hormones — including all three estrogens, testosterone, and progesterone. Issues such as elevated **Androstenedione** may indicate metabolic dysfunction and/or ovarian cysts, which contribute to fertility issues.

① RECOMMENDED LABS

ACCESS MEDICAL LABS

OpenDx Saliva Hormone Supreme

ULTA LAB TESTS · COMBO PANEL

Luteinizing Hormone (LH) & Follicle-Stimulating Hormone (FSH)

ZRT LABORATORY

Cardiometabolic Panel

② THE HORMONE KIT

HOMEOPATHIC · USE PER LAB RESULTS

DR. DALE'S NUFEM #1

Homeopathic Progesterone Topical Spray (IF PROGESTERONE IS LOW)

> DOSE 1–4 sprays on the inner arm, Days 12–28 of your cycle. 5 days on, 2 days off.

Use if progesterone is low or needs balancing.

> If progesterone is **high**, use the Original Hormone-Free formulas instead.

DR. DALE'S NUFEM #2

Homeopathic Estrogen Topical Spray (IF ESTROGEN IS LOW)

> DOSE 1–2 sprays, Days 1–28 of your cycle. 5 days on, 2 days off.

Use if estrogen(s) are low.

> If estrogen is **high**, use the Original Hormone-Free formulas instead.

DR. DALE'S NUFEM #3

Homeopathic Testosterone Spray (IF TESTOSTERONE IS LOW)

DOSE 1–4 sprays on the inner arm, Days 12–28 of your cycle. 5 days on, 2 days off.

Use if testosterone is low.

> If testosterone is **high**, use the Original Hormone-Free formulas instead.

DR. DALE'S

Bio Age Reverse Drops

DOSE 5 drops under the tongue, Monday–Friday.

Supports overall hormone balance across the endocrine system and completes the hormone kit.

DR. DALE'S

MBM/NER Female #13

DOSE 5 drops under the tongue, Monday–Friday.

Supports overall hormone balance for the female endocrine system specifically, and completes the hormone kit.

③ OVARIAN & METABOLIC SUPPORT

SKIN NATUROPATHIC

Hormonal Breakouts Female

DOSE 2–5 capsules, 3 times daily with meals.

Balances ovarian function and hormonal profiles in women prone to ovarian cysts, excess androgens, and metabolic dysfunction that may impact their ability to conceive and carry to term.

⚠ STOP IF YOU BECOME PREGNANT

DR. DALE'S

Full Body Detoxification Kit

DOSE 3 caps each of Kidney Pro, Liver Pro & Whole-Body Immune Pro with each meal daily. 1–2 capsules of Colon Pro with each meal daily. Reduce the dose if diarrhea develops.

Begin detoxification 5 days on, 2 days off. Continue for 3–6 months.

⚠ STOP IMMEDIATELY IF YOU BECOME PREGNANT

④ EGG QUALITY & FOUNDATIONAL SUPPORT

PURE ENCAPSULATIONS

Ubiquinol 100 mg

> **DOSE** 400–600 mg per day (4–6 capsules).

This antioxidant supports egg quality and health.

DR. DALE'S

Nano-Ionic Iodine

> **DOSE** 30 drops daily in water.

BIOTICS RESEARCH

Fe-Zyme

> **DOSE** 1 tablet in the AM.

PENDULUM

GLP-1 Probiotic Pro

> **DOSE** 1 capsule daily with the first meal.

VITAL NUTRIENTS

Ultra-Pure Fish Oil 700

> **DOSE** 1 capsule daily.

BIOTICS RESEARCH

Lipoic Acid Plus

> **DOSE** 1 capsule 3 times daily with meals.

BIOTICS RESEARCH

Bio Protect Plus

> **DOSE** 1 capsule 3 times daily with meals.

BIOTICS RESEARCH

CLA

> **DOSE** 1 capsule twice daily with meals.

⑤ RECOMMENDED PEPTIDES

REJUVATIDE PEPTIDES

REJUVATIDE PEPTIDES

Kisspeptin-10 — 5 mg

> DOSE Reconstitute with 2 mL bacteriostatic water. Inject 2–6 units in the AM, daily or every other day, during the late follicular phase (often cycle days ~8–14, depending on follicle development).

Repeat every cycle until ovulation occurs, or until FSH and LH come into range.

> Not needed if you are ovulating normally, or already have in-range LH and FSH.

PEPTIDE SCIENCE

Gonadorelin — 5 mg

> DOSE Reconstitute with 2 mL bacteriostatic water. 4–8 units morning and evening on the 3–7 days leading up to ovulation, into the abdomen or thigh.

Boosts native LH/FSH signaling. Repeat each cycle until ovulation occurs.

> Not needed if you are already ovulating and have proper LH and FSH levels.

REJUVATIDE PEPTIDES · GLP-1 FAMILY

Metabolic Peptide (Sema, Tirz, Reta, Maz) — single, dual or triple agonist

> DOSE Reconstitute with 1 mL bacteriostatic water. 1–3 units once weekly on the same day. 8 weeks on, 2 weeks off.

This is a tiny **micro-dose** used for insulin sensitivity rather than weight loss, and supports proper metabolic function and blood sugar metabolism. If you also need to lose weight, you can go up to 25 units and cycle 12 weeks on, 4 weeks off.

⑥ PROTOCOL NOTES

1. **Confirm whether you are ovulating.** Please confirm with a medical doctor whether or not you are ovulating — this is important. Home ovulation test kits are an acceptable option, but medical confirmation is preferred.

2. **Check for cysts and androgens.** It is important to know if you have cystic ovaries and elevated androstenedione. Cysts can be confirmed by ultrasound; androstenedione and cortisol levels need to be assessed with the saliva test.

3. **LH, FSH & insulin resistance.** Know whether LH and FSH are low so they can be addressed. Insulin resistance is another key piece — it can lead to elevated androgens, which cause issues with ovulation and fertility.

4. **Why progesterone is timed.** The homeopathic recommendations are designed to return your hormones to a normal cycle. Using the Progest formula only in the second half of the cycle mimics what the body should do post-ovulation.

IF YOU CONCEIVE BUT CANNOT CARRY TO TERM

Progesterone is important for the first 13 weeks. If you conceive, you may need to take a progesterone replacement (HRT) during this time, until the placenta is able to take over and make progesterone.

⑦ STOP ALL STIMULANTS

1. **Caffeine must be 100% avoided** on this protocol, or it will stop the homeopathy from working. Please wean yourself off by 25% less every week. Coffee substitutes can be found at www.Teeccino.com.

2. **Mint** — such as in tea and essential oils on the skin — should be used in moderation, as mint may interfere with homeopathic remedies.

3. **Sugar is also a stimulant** and should be avoided.

This protocol is provided for educational purposes and is intended for patients under the care of a qualified practitioner. It is not a substitute for individualized medical advice, diagnosis, or treatment. Confirm ovulation and evaluate hormone, androgen, and metabolic status with appropriate testing before beginning. Several items must be stopped immediately upon a confirmed or suspected pregnancy, as noted. Do not begin, stop, or adjust any hormone, peptide, or supplement without consulting your provider — particularly if you are pregnant, trying to conceive, nursing, taking medications, or managing a medical condition.

CLINICAL PROTOCOL · 100% NATURAL

Low Testosterone in Men

BY **DIANA M. DRAKE, BCTN** · DMD NATURAL MEDICINE

To properly address Low-T in men, it is important to determine the root cause: is it from poor signaling from the **HPG axis** (hypothalamic-pituitary-gonadal), or have the testes physically begun to shut down? An ongoing blood test that looks at both free and bound testosterone is acceptable as a follow-up; the saliva test is recommended initially to examine potential estrogenic imbalances and adrenal cortisol patterns.

⚠ **First, identify the root cause.**
If the testes have physically shut down, **HRT is the only option**. If the issue is poor signaling, it can often be corrected — the protocol below is worth trying first in that case.

① RECOMMENDED LABS

ACCESS MEDICAL LABS
OpenDx Saliva Hormone Supreme

BLOOD PANEL
LH & FSH

② HOW TO INTERPRET THE PATTERN

PATTERN	LIKELY CAUSE
Low testosterone + **high LH/FSH**	**Primary hypogonadism** — the testes are not responding.
Low testosterone + **low or normal LH/FSH**	**Secondary hypogonadism** — hypothalamus / pituitary suppression.
Normal testosterone + **low LH**	**External testosterone or androgen suppression.**

③ SUPPLEMENTS FOR LOW-T IN MEN

DR. DALE'S

Homeopathic Testosterone Male

DOSE 5 drops in the AM & PM, Monday–Friday only. No caffeine.

DR. DALE'S

Bio Age Reverse Drops

DOSE 5 drops under the tongue twice daily, AM & PM, on an empty stomach. Monday–Friday only. No caffeine.

DR. DALE'S

MBM Male Tincture

DOSE 5 drops under the tongue twice daily, AM & PM, on an empty stomach. Monday–Friday only. No caffeine.

AMAZON OR DIRECT

EPIC-T

DOSE 1 capsule daily.

DR. DALE'S

Full Body Detoxification Kit

DOSE 3 caps each of Kidney Pro, Liver Pro & Whole-Body Immune Pro with each meal daily. 1–2 capsules of Colon Pro with each meal daily. Reduce the dose if diarrhea develops.

Begin detoxification 5 days on, 2 days off. Repeat the detox for 3–6 months.

DR. DALE'S

Optimal Multi-Pro

DOSE 1–2 caps daily with the first meal of the day.

Supports adrenal balance with vitamins and adaptogens.

> If cortisol was severely out of balance, also add **Dr. Dale's Adaptogen Pro**, taken during the times of day your cortisol was ow or high.

④ RECOMMENDED PEPTIDES

REJUVATIDE PEPTIDES

PEPTIDE SCIENCE

Gonadorelin — 5 mg

> DOSE Reconstitute with 1 mL bacteriostatic water. 4–8 units once or twice daily, AM & PM. Cycle 8–12 weeks on, 4 weeks off.

Corrects signaling from the HPG axis that tells the male testes to make testosterone. **For this to work, the testes must still be functional.**

> Re-test testosterone during the off cycle.

REJUVATIDE PEPTIDES

Tesamorelin — 10 mg

> DOSE Reconstitute with 2 mL bacteriostatic water. 100–200 units once daily, in the evening before bed, for 12–16 weeks, then rest for 4 weeks.

An upstream peptide that works on signaling from the glandular system. If the male testes have shut down, this peptide will not improve the situation.

⚠ DO NOT USE WITH A KNOWN PITUITARY TUMOR

⑤ PROTOCOL NOTES

STOP ALL STIMULANTS

1. **Caffeine must be 100% avoided** on this protocol, or it will stop the homeopathy from working. Please wean yourself off by 25% less every week. Coffee substitutes can be found at www.Teeccino.com.
2. **Mint** — such as in tea and essential oils on the skin — should be used in moderation, as mint may interfere with homeopathic remedies.
3. **Sugar is also a stimulant** and should be avoided.

This protocol is provided for educational purposes and is intended for patients under the care of a qualified practitioner. It is not a substitute for individualized medical advice, diagnosis, or treatment. Testosterone status should be evaluated with appropriate saliva and blood testing to determine the root cause before beginning. Do not use Tesamorelin with a known pituitary tumor. Do not begin, stop, or adjust any hormone, peptide, or supplement without consulting your provider, particularly if you are managing a medical condition.

CLINICAL PROTOCOL · 100% NATURAL

Erectile Support in Men

BY **DIANA M. DRAKE, BCTN** · DMD NATURAL MEDICINE

> First, refer to the **Low Testosterone in Men** protocol to test for testosterone levels and assess testicle function. If testosterone is low, that will need to be corrected first.

⚠ **Manage blood pressure first — naturally.**
If your blood pressure is high, or you are on blood pressure medication, it must be properly managed **before** implementing this protocol. The root of the blood pressure issue needs to be resolved — not masked by a drug. Please reference the **Blood Pressure Management** protocol and get it in balance PRIOR to doing this protocol for proper healing and results.

① RECOMMENDED LABS

ACCESS MEDICAL LABS

OpenDx Supreme Saliva Hormone Test

BLOOD PANEL

LH & FSH

Helps determine whether the issue is poor signaling versus testes unable to produce.

FOLLOW-UP TESTING

An ongoing blood test that looks at both free and bound testosterone is acceptable as a follow-up. The saliva test is recommended initially to examine potential estrogenic imbalances and adrenal cortisol patterns.

② HOW TO INTERPRET THE PATTERN

PATTERN	LIKELY CAUSE
Low testosterone + **high LH/FSH**	**Primary hypogonadism** — the testes are not responding.
Low testosterone + **low or normal LH/FSH**	**Secondary hypogonadism** — hypothalamus / pituitary suppression.
Normal testosterone + **low LH**	**External testosterone or androgen suppression.**

③ SUPPLEMENTS

AMAZON

EPIC-T

DOSE 1 capsule before activity.

DR. DALE'S

Oxygen Pro

DOSE 20 drops 3× daily in **mineralized** water — AM, afternoon & PM.

If extra minerals / electrolytes are not added, the oxygen will not properly absorb. Add about ½ teaspoon of salt to each glass of water, 3× daily.

RE-SYNC RECOVERY

Nitric Oxide Blend

DOSE 1 scoop with water, smoothie, yogurt or oats, once daily.

Ideal times to take it: about 1 hour pre-workout, 1 hour post-workout, or 1 hour before bed.

④ RECOMMENDED PEPTIDES

REJUVATIDE PEPTIDES

REJUVATIDE PEPTIDES · SEXUAL WELLNESS

PT-141 — 10 mg

DOSE Reconstitute with 2 mL bacteriostatic water. Use 10 or more units prior to activity, or daily, and see how you feel — you may increase as needed.

⚠ DO NOT USE IF ANY OF THE FOLLOWING APPLY

- Unmanaged high blood pressure.
- Cardiovascular conditions such as hypertension / high blood pressure.
- In combination with erectile dysfunction drugs.
- Not advisable to use while drinking alcohol.

This peptide may also be taken via nasal application instead of injection: reconstitute with saline solution and load it into a nasal spray bottle, or source a pre-made nasal spray online.

REJUVATIDE PEPTIDES

Oxytocin — 2 mg

DOSE Reconstitute with 2 mL bacteriostatic water. Use 10–20 units 30 minutes prior to sexual activity, as needed.

This peptide may also be taken via nasal application instead of injection: reconstitute with saline solution and load it into a nasal spray bottle, or source a pre-made nasal spray online.

⑤ PROTOCOL NOTES

STOP ALL STIMULANTS

1. **Caffeine must be 100% avoided** on this protocol, or it will stop the homeopathy from working. Please wean yourself off by 25% less every week. Coffee substitutes can be found at www.Teeccino.com.

2. **Mint** — such as in tea and essential oils on the skin — should be used in moderation, as mint may interfere with homeopathic remedies.

3. **Sugar is also a stimulant** and should be avoided.

This protocol is provided for educational purposes and is intended for patients under the care of a qualified practitioner. It is not a substitute for individualized medical advice, diagnosis, or treatment. Address low testosterone and blood pressure first, as noted. Do not use PT-141 with unmanaged high blood pressure, cardiovascular conditions, erectile dysfunction medications, or alcohol. Do not begin, stop, or adjust any hormone, peptide, or supplement without consulting your provider, particularly if you are managing a medical condition.

CLINICAL PROTOCOL · 100% NATURAL

Low Libido & Sexual Interest

Low libido & lack of sexual interest — for men & women

BY **DIANA M. DRAKE, BCTN** · DMD NATURAL MEDICINE

① RECOMMENDED PEPTIDES

REJUVATIDE PEPTIDES

REJUVATIDE PEPTIDES · THE "LOVE HORMONE"

Oxytocin — 2 mg

DOSE Reconstitute with 2 mL bacteriostatic water. 10–20 units, 30 minutes prior to sexual activity, as needed.

Known as the "Love Hormone," this peptide helps increase the body's native oxytocin production.

REJUVATIDE PEPTIDES · SEXUAL DESIRE & AROUSAL

PT-141 — 10 mg

DOSE **WOMEN:** 10 units AM or PM as needed.
MEN: begin with 10 units and increase to 20–40 units AM or PM as needed.
Inject sub-Q in the stomach or outer thigh. Reconstitute with 2 mL bacteriostatic water.

Known as the sexual desire and arousal peptide.

⚠ DO NOT USE IF YOU HAVE ELEVATED BLOOD PRESSURE

② HERBAL LIBIDO SUPPORT

NATURE'S SUNSHINE

X-Action Reloaded FOR MEN

DOSE 2 caps nightly before bed.

NATURE'S SUNSHINE

Women's X-Action Reloaded FOR WOMEN

DOSE 2 caps with a meal, 3 times daily.

This protocol is provided for educational purposes and is intended for patients under the care of a qualified practitioner. It is not a substitute for individualized medical advice, diagnosis, or treatment. Do not use PT-141 if you have elevated blood pressure. Do not begin, stop, or adjust any peptide or supplement without consulting your provider, particularly if you are managing a medical condition or taking medications.

A BIOHACKING PROTOCOL · 100% NATURAL

Reverse Aging

Antioxidant, cellular & longevity support

BY **DIANA M. DRAKE, BCTN** · DMD NATURAL MEDICINE

① RECOMMENDED LABS

OPTIONAL

Labs are optional but can provide incredible insight into your body's aging process. Ideally, run these before the protocol and test again in 90 days to see improvements — at which point you can decide whether to repeat the protocol.

TRUDIAGNOSTIC

TruAge

A comprehensive test that helps you understand your biological age, with a variety of reports that measure different aspects of your health and compare them to your chronological age.

GENOMIC TESTING

Methylation Genomics

Looks at specific variations in your genes that can affect your body's methylation pathway. Methylation is critical in many biological processes, including energy production and mood regulation.

CELLULAR AGING MARKER

Telomere Length Test

Measures the length of your telomeres — the protective caps on the ends of your chromosomes that naturally shorten with age. Telomere length is used as a marker of cellular aging.

② SUPPLEMENTS

DR. DALE'S

Bio Age Erase — Vitamin C, Collagen & Silica Powder

DOSE 1 scoop 3× daily in a glass of water or juice.

Antioxidants are the key to anti-aging — the fight against oxidative stress and oxidative aging. This supplement has no filler, sweetener, or added flavoring; it has a naturally acrid, chalky taste, so it may be best taken with a fresh-pressed juice.

PURE ENCAPSULATIONS

Resveratrol EXTRA

> **DOSE** 1 capsule daily with a meal.

Resveratrol is a powerful antioxidant that fights oxidative stress and free-radical damage.

DR. DALE'S

Nano-Ionic Iodine

> **DOSE** 30 drops daily in water. If deficient (as most are), you can start with a loading dose of 90 drops per day.

Iodine is crucial for proper hormone function in men and women. Dr. Dale's iodine is decolorized so as not to stain.

③ RECOMMENDED PEPTIDES & INJECTABLES

REJUVATIDE PEPTIDES

REJUVATIDE PEPTIDES

NAD+ — 500 mg

> **DOSE** Reconstitute the bottle all the way up to the bottle neck. Inject 50–200 units sub-Q into the fatty tissue of the stomach, thighs, or back of the arm, AM or PM, twice weekly for 2–3 weeks.

Rest for a week, then repeat the cycle. You may also decrease to a foundational support of 25 units twice weekly, after you have been on the 50-unit dose for some time.

⚠ CONTRAINDICATED WITH CERTAIN ACTIVE CANCERS — DO NOT USE WITH ACTIVE CANCER UNLESS CLEARED BY A MEDICAL DOCTOR

REJUVATIDE PEPTIDES

MOTS-c — 10 mg

> **DOSE** Reconstitute with 3 mL bacteriostatic water. Inject 100 units 3×/week in ongoing cycles; rest as needed. Sub-Q into fatty tissue of the stomach, thighs, or back of the arm.

REJUVATIDE PEPTIDES

Epithalon — 10 mg

> **DOSE** Reconstitute with 1 mL bacteriostatic water. Inject 100 units — an entire syringe full — for 10 days straight, in the PM. This is one bottle per day. Sub-Q into fatty tissue of the stomach, thighs, or back of the arm.

REJUVATIDE PEPTIDES · BPC + TB-500 + GHK-CU

GLOW Blend

> **DOSE** Reconstitute with 3.5 mL bacteriostatic water (less water makes it more potent, but you'll go through the peptide quicker). Dose once daily, 8 weeks on, 2 weeks off. For a highly aesthetic protocol (skin results): up to 80 units. Maintenance dose: 20–30 units every other day.

This protocol is provided for educational purposes and is intended for patients under the care of a qualified practitioner. It is not a substitute for individualized medical advice, diagnosis, or treatment. NAD+ is contraindicated with certain active cancers — do not use it with active cancer unless cleared by a medical doctor. Do not begin, stop, or adjust any peptide, injectable, or supplement without consulting your provider, particularly if you are managing a medical condition or taking medications.

HORMONE REPLACEMENT THERAPY

HRT Protocol for Women

For women who: cease to have a monthly cycle · fertility · low-hormone fatigue · hormones not responding to homeopathy

BY **DIANA M. DRAKE, BCTN** · DMD NATURAL MEDICINE

① RECOMMENDED LABS

Access Medical Labs — OpenDx Saliva Hormone with 4× Cortisol. If hormones are low in any of the areas below, you can use the corresponding remedies as long as you continue to monitor hormone levels every 90 days. Homeopathy is still recommended to harmonize the HRT and help balance the body.

② TARGETED HRT — BY LOW HORMONE

IF PROGESTERONE IS LOW

QUICKSILVER SCIENTIFIC · TOPICAL

Pro Progesterone

DOSE **CYCLING WOMEN:** 2 pumps AM & PM, days 14–28.
NO LONGER CYCLING: daily.

↻ RE-TEST HORMONES IN 6 WEEKS

IF TESTOSTERONE IS LOW

BY PRESCRIPTION · DMD TELEHEALTH

Testosterone Replacement Therapy

Requires HRT from a medical doctor (testosterone replacement therapy). Use the **DMD Telehealth service** at www.DMDNaturalMedicine.com.

IF ESTROGEN(S) ARE LOW

QUICKSILVER SCIENTIFIC

Pro Estrogen Formulas

Pro Estriol

Pro Estradiol

Pro B-Estrogen — contains both estrogen types

DOSE 1 pump, 1–2 times daily.

↻ RE-TEST HORMONES IN 6 WEEKS

IF DHEA IS LOW

DHEA — 5 mg

Pure Encapsulations DHEA 5 mg — 1 capsule in the AM.

— OR —

Quicksilver Scientific Oral Liquid DHEA 5 mg — 1 pump in the mouth.

> **First** see if your body converts this into other hormones before you begin using progesterone and estrogens.

IF ALL HORMONES ARE LOW

PURE ENCAPSULATIONS

Pregnenolone — 10 mg

> DOSE 1 capsule in the AM.

First see if your body converts this into progesterone and estrogens before taking the topicals.

> If it doesn't convert and DHEA is known to be low, try using DHEA instead. You do not need to do both — try one, then the other.

③ TO HARMONIZE THE PROTOCOL

DR. DALE'S

MenoGel

> DOSE **IF CYCLING:** 1 pump AM & PM, days 14–28 of your cycle. 5 days on, 2 days off.
> **IF NO LONGER CYCLING:** 1–2 pumps AM & PM, Monday–Friday every week.

④ SUPPLEMENTS

DR. DALE'S

Nano-Ionic Iodine

> DOSE 30 drops daily in water.

Iodine is imperative for proper hormone function in both men and women, and most are deficient — especially women.

⑤ PROTOCOL NOTES

This protocol is provided as a backup for those who, for any reason, choose to or need to implement HRT to reach their goals. You can also get HRT from a medical doctor using our Virtual Telehealth service at www.DMDNaturalMedicine.com.

This protocol involves hormone replacement therapy and is provided for educational purposes for patients under the care of a qualified practitioner. It is not a substitute for individualized medical advice, diagnosis, or treatment. Hormone levels must be tested before starting and monitored every 90 days (with a 6-week recheck after starting a new hormone). Do not begin, stop, or adjust any hormone, precursor, or supplement without consulting your provider — particularly if you are pregnant, trying to conceive, nursing, taking medications, or managing a medical condition.

MENOPAUSE HRT ADJUNCT PROTOCOL

HRT Boost Add-On

BY **DIANA M. DRAKE, BCTN** · DMD NATURAL MEDICINE

① HOW TO USE THIS ADD-ON

Take all the recommendations from the **Natural Menopause Protocol** first. Then, if needed, you can add hormone replacement therapy (HRT) based on your lab results.

⚠ **Do not take HRT without proper saliva hormone test monitoring.**
Bio-identical hormones are dosed to your labs and re-tested over time. Never begin or adjust HRT without testing.

② RECOMMENDED HRT

BIO-IDENTICAL · PER LAB RESULTS

PURE ENCAPSULATIONS

DHEA — 5–25 mg, oral (IF DHEA IS LOW)

Use this precursor **only if your labs show DHEA is low.** Dosed to your saliva panel — start at the low end and adjust with retesting.

PURE ENCAPSULATIONS

Pregnenolone — 5–20 mg, oral (IF DHEA IS NOT LOW)

If your DHEA is not low, Pregnenolone is the precursor option to try instead. Dose to your labs; begin low and titrate as directed.

QUICKSILVER SCIENTIFIC

Topical Bio-Identical Progesterone

DOSE ¼ to 1 pump daily, Monday–Friday.

Applied topically. Adjust within the range according to your labs and symptoms.

QUICKSILVER SCIENTIFIC

Bio-Identical Estriol & Estradiol

FORM Available as a combination, or as individual formulas.

Estrogen support dosed to your saliva hormone results. Your practitioner will determine the combination and strength.

BY PRESCRIPTION · TELEMEDICINE

Testosterone

Available only through our online telemedicine service, as this is a controlled substance requiring a prescription.

⚠ CONTROLLED SUBSTANCE · PRESCRIPTION REQUIRED

③ LIVER SUPPORT

DR. DALE'S

Liver Pro

DOSE 2 caps with each meal daily, to help the liver process the HRT.

Continue taking this after you complete the full-body detox in the Natural Menopause Protocol.

This protocol is provided for educational purposes and is intended for patients under the care of a qualified practitioner. It is not a substitute for individualized medical advice, diagnosis, or treatment. Hormone replacement therapy must be guided by saliva hormone testing and ongoing monitoring. Do not begin, stop, or adjust any hormone, precursor, or supplement without consulting your provider — particularly if you are pregnant or nursing, taking medications, or managing a medical condition.

CHAPTER 2

Weight Loss, Metabolism & Cholesterol

According to recent statistics and Dr. Casey Means (Good Energy Book), over 93% of Americans have some form of metabolic dysfunction, defined as a pathological state where normal metabolic pathways - such as glucose regulation, lipid metabolism, insulin signaling, and mitochondrial energy production are disrupted.

Metabolic function can show up as:

- Diagnosed diabetes (A1C over 6.5)
- Diagnosed pre-diabetic (A1C above 5.2 according to functional range)
- Insulin resistance (cells cannot "see" insulin properly leading to elevated blood sugar and the body storing sugar as fat)
- Overweight or stubborn belly fat at any age that is resistant to diet and exercise
- Elevated blood sugar
- Elevated triglycerides
- Low HDL ("good") cholesterol
- Chronic low-grade inflammation
- Mitochondrial inefficiency or oxidative stress
- Obesity
- Non-alcoholic fatty liver disease
- Cardiovascular disease
- PCOS (Poly-Cystic Ovarian Syndrome)
- Painful and severe periods in young women
- Skipping periods in young women

Looking at the blood sugar puzzle piece first, western medicine ranges for A1C are 5.3 - 5.6 for insulin resistance and 5.7 - 6.4 for pre-diabetics. Functional ranges are a lot tighter - and more accurate. A1C in a normal blood sugar profile should be 4.8-5.2. A1C above 5.2 indicates your body is handling blood sugar poorly, yet your doctor may not mention it because according to standard ranges, you would still be "in range". This misunderstanding in blood sugar ranges is exactly why insulin resistance is wildly under-diagnosed in western medicine.

Imagine hearing that your blood sugar is "normal", but you have high cholesterol and issues with your menstrual cycle, acne, stubborn belly fat... yet you are being told "everything is fine". Blood sugar ranges are also inaccurate from a functional view. Western medicine allows you to go up to 99 on your fasting blood sugar levels, when you should really be 75-85 for the optimal range. In 2024, the FDA changed the law to allow continuous glucose monitors to be sold over the counter. Before this time, you couldn't even get one unless you were diagnosed with diabetics, and then you had to have a prescription for a monitor from your doctor. That meant there was no way to monitor your blood sugar proactively, unless you wanted to prick your finger after every single meal. You can now get over the counter "constant" blood sugar monitors that provide continuous feedback on your levels. A brand like Stello is available on Amazon for $99 per month. I recommend using one for 90 days to really track which foods spike your blood sugar and to see how the protocol(s) below help you over time. If you like your results, you can use the blood sugar monitor for a longer term as well.

When it comes to menopause, weight gain is typically the primary complaint as it begins around perimenopause and worsens as you progress into menopause. Weight gain is due to an increase in insulin resistance as we age - and it happens to men too. Insulin resistance is a metabolic condition in which the body's cells no longer respond appropriately to insulin, forcing the pancreas to produce more to keep your blood sugar stable. Over time, this leads to elevated insulin levels, disrupted blood sugar control, and increased risk for prediabetes, type 2 diabetes, and metabolic dysfunction. In other words, your body is now storing carbs and sugar as fat. Aging men and women tend to benefit immensely from going on a keto diet. When the body is in ketosis, it switches from burning sugar (carbohydrates) as a fuel to burning fat.

Now I have had many clients who love using the keto diet and the benefits that it has on their metabolism and weight control. Eating keto means you only eat protein and high-fat foods to switch your body's metabolic process. Fruit, dairy, bread, and most carbs are eliminated. Eating keto is incredibly restrictive and takes a lot of willpower. Those of my clients who do it long term thrive and absolutely love how they feel and look. But the reality is that for most people, it is not a sustainable way to eat - especially if you have a family to feed.

One of the new and popular weight loss crazes of 2026 is the Ozempic and GLP-1 drug choices. Losing weight at a rapid pace on these medications causes now-known side effects, including a reduction in bone density, saggy skin, malnutrition, and the inability to have healthy bowel movements. Additionally, you must stay on it forever, or the weight comes back. Losing 20+ pounds in 30 days is not a safe rate of weight loss. Closer to 2 pounds a week is reasonable and healthier.

You will see that my weight-loss protocols do call for a GLP-1 Peptide to address insulin resistance and reduce food cravings. Benefiting from this peptide without the horrible side effects is as simple as a dose reduction, which we call "microdosing". Unfortunately, weight loss clinics have been grossly overdosing people on these GLP medications, giving GLP drugs and peptides a bad reputation. The reality is that at the proper dose, GLP-1 is incredible at balancing your blood sugar and helping with healthy, sustainable weight loss.

There is a strong metabolic connection to cardiovascular disease, the #1 killer of men & women in America today. This makes it very important to understand the metabolic component as a root cause in these cases. Using a statin drug to lower your cholesterol is not good enough in attempting to treat and prevent cardiovascular disease. I would know, because my mother passed away of a heart attack in 2007 with perfectly "in range" cholesterol levels due to being on a statin drug. Statin Drugs are designed to change how your liver processes fat, resulting in a lower distribution of cholesterol into your arteries. Statin drugs may "lower" your cholesterol levels, but here is what it will not do :

- Significantly lower inflammatory markers like C-Reactive Protein and Homocysteine levels (though it may lower some).
- Stop blood clots from forming by breaking down Fibrin. Fibrin is the protein found in blood - forming long, insoluble strands creating a mesh that forms a blood clot. Blood clots are important if you cut your skin as they are part of the body's repair process to stop bleeding - but not something we want happening in the blood vessels. Blood clots can obstruct circulation, leading to strokes, heart attacks, and other cardiovascular or neurological complications.
- Provide crucial antioxidant support for cardiovascular and blood vessel tissue (CoQ10), in fact it will actually suppress the production of Co-Q10.
- Provide the heart and vascular system with basic essential nutrients like potassium and magnesium. This is very important as the heart is electrical and requires certain electrolytes for balance.
- Prevent calcium deposits from forming plaque.
- Stop the arterial walls from hardening (arteriosclerosis).

Just because your cholesterol is "high" doesn't necessarily correlate with being overweight. In fact, people who are healthy and look to be in shape can and do still suffer from this imbalance. It's not something you can "see" and don't assume it to only be on an overweight person. To properly check both your lipid panel, blood sugar levels and inflammatory markers, I recommend the ZRT Cardiometabolic Panel which is an easy at home finger-prick blood spot sample.

The point I would really like you to take home here is that you need to look at all these biomarkers to properly assess metabolism. When you fully understand the whole picture - you can now act confidently with the proper protocol. My protocols that follow will address metabolic dysfunction as a root cause. If you're found not to have metabolic dysfunction, which I rarely see in my practice, I also provide a general protocol for weight loss that may work for your case instead. Keep in mind that if you have a thyroid issue, that needs to be corrected as an underlying condition - which I address in Chapter 11, Thyroid Protocols.

CLINICAL PROTOCOL · 100% NATURAL

Weight Gain / Cannot Lose Weight

Metabolic & blood-sugar support for stubborn weight

BY **DIANA M. DRAKE, BCTN** · DMD NATURAL MEDICINE

① RECOMMENDED LABS

ZRT LABORATORY

Cardiometabolic Test Kit

② SUPPLEMENTS

DR. DALE'S

Berberine Pro

DOSE 1 cap with each meal, for blood sugar balance.

Berberine lowers blood sugar and improves A1C primarily by activating **AMPK** (AMP-activated protein kinase), the cell's master metabolic switch. When AMPK is activated, it:

- Increases glucose uptake into muscle cells
- Reduces hepatic glucose production (less sugar released by the liver)
- Improves insulin receptor sensitivity
- Enhances mitochondrial function and fatty acid oxidation
- Slows carbohydrate breakdown in the gut (via α-glucosidase inhibition)

Together, these actions reduce fasting glucose, lower post-meal spikes, and gradually improve A1C.

DR. DALE'S

Nano-Ionic Iodine — or Bio-Iodine (stronger)

DOSE Nano-Ionic Iodine: 30 drops daily in water.

Iodine is crucial for proper hormone function in men and women.

> If deficient, use the stronger **Bio-Iodine** caps.

③ RECOMMENDED PEPTIDES

REJUVATIDE PEPTIDES

REJUVATIDE PEPTIDES · GLP-1 FAMILY

Metabolic Peptide — single, dual or triple agonist, 10 mg

> DOSE Reconstitute with 1 mL bacteriostatic water. 10–25 units once weekly, or every 5 days. 12 weeks on, 4 weeks off. Increase by 5 units per week until you feel the "food chatter" turn off and appetite decrease.

This is a **microdose** — the idea is not to starve yourself, but to eat smaller, healthier meals while managing blood sugar. GLP-1 peptides regulate metabolic and digestive function by signaling between the gut, pancreas, and brain; increased insulin sensitivity lets the body better use food as fuel rather than storing it as fat. GLP-1 "drugs" taken at high doses are dangerous, but a microdose of the peptide can be safe and effective without creating reliance.

REJUVATIDE PEPTIDES · GROWTH-HORMONE SECRETAGOGUE

CJC-1295 + Ipamorelin — 10 mg blend

> DOSE **FASTING CARDIO:** 10–15 units pre-workout.
> **LIFTING WEIGHTS:** 10–25 units post-workout, then fast 90 minutes before eating.
> **NOT WORKING OUT:** take in the evening before bed.
> 5 days a week is ideal. Cycle 8 weeks on, 4 weeks off. Reconstitute with 2 mL bacteriostatic water.

Helps maintain lean muscle mass by encouraging your body to secrete more of its own Human Growth Hormone; also helps with recovery and sleep. It is normal to feel a "niacin flush" type response — in high-histamine individuals this may be intense.

> Tesamorelin and Sermorelin are also good growth-hormone secretagogues for those more sensitive to this blend — keep them in mind as alternatives if necessary.

⚠ GROWTH-FACTOR PEPTIDES ARE NOT RECOMMENDED WITH ACTIVE CANCER

④ PROTOCOL NOTES

LIFESTYLE

Avoiding carbs and sugar is extremely helpful for weight loss, as is getting some form of aerobic activity. Light cardio and light weightlifting are great for burning fat and building lean muscle. If you don't enjoy the gym, try a Pilates class or another group class at an intensity level you enjoy and can commit to a few days a week.

CLINICAL PROTOCOL · 100% NATURAL

Blood Sugar Imbalance / Insulin Issues

Metabolic & insulin-sensitivity support

BY **DIANA M. DRAKE, BCTN** · DMD NATURAL MEDICINE

① RECOMMENDED LABS

ZRT LABORATORY

Cardiometabolic Panel

HOW TO READ IT

Functional A1C is 4.9–5.2 — anything above 5.2 may indicate poor blood sugar handling, even when standard lab ranges call it "normal." If you have been diagnosed as pre-diabetic or with type 2 diabetes, your sugar levels are dangerously high and are negatively affecting your health.

For your follow-up panel, you can run only a glucose & A1C panel if those were the only values elevated. If your cholesterol is also elevated, please see the **Cholesterol** protocol.

⚠ **Always fast before blood sugar testing.**
You must always be fasting when taking any kind of blood sugar test, or the results will not be accurate.

② SUPPLEMENTS

DR. DALE'S

Berberine Pro

DOSE 1 capsule with each meal.

DR. DALE'S

Bio Age Reverse Drops

DOSE 5 drops in the AM & PM, Monday–Friday only. No caffeine.

③ RECOMMENDED PEPTIDES

REJUVATIDE PEPTIDES

REJUVATIDE PEPTIDES · GLP-1 FAMILY

Metabolic Peptide — single, dual or triple agonist, 10 mg

> DOSE Reconstitute with 1 mL bacteriostatic water. Inject 2.5–5 units weekly on the same day of the week. 12 weeks on, 4 weeks off.

Works on insulin sensitivity. The purpose of this dose is **blood sugar management, not weight loss.**

↻ RE-CHECK GLUCOSE & A1C EVERY 6 WEEKS — ADJUST DOSE TO KEEP IT BALANCED

④ DIETARY RECOMMENDATIONS

1. It is very important to **avoid processed grains and sugar** if you have metabolic dysfunction in the form of elevated blood sugar.

2. If you are going to eat grains, **organic whole grains** are ideal — in a bowl, or with a meal as a side alongside protein.

This protocol is provided for educational purposes and is intended for patients under the care of a qualified practitioner. It is not a substitute for individualized medical advice, diagnosis, or treatment. Blood sugar testing must always be done fasting. Do not begin, stop, or adjust any peptide, supplement, or diabetes medication without consulting your provider, particularly if you are pre-diabetic, diabetic, or otherwise managing a medical condition.

CLINICAL PROTOCOL · 100% NATURAL

Elevated Cholesterol & Inflammatory Biomarkers

Lipid, vascular & inflammation support

BY **DIANA M. DRAKE, BCTN** · DMD NATURAL MEDICINE

① RECOMMENDED LABS

ZRT LABORATORY

Cardiometabolic Panel

FUNCTIONAL RANGES — STRICTER THAN THE LAB

A1C TARGET	FASTING GLUCOSE TARGET
4.8 – 5.2	**75 – 85 mg/dL**

If you are above these, even though the lab shows "in range," we recognize this as out of range in functional medicine — meaning it needs to be addressed. Western medical ranges let you go as high as 5.6 before you are told you are pre-diabetic. This is not the school of thought in naturopathic medicine, and it is why metabolic dysfunction is so often overlooked and not properly diagnosed by Western medicine.

↻ RE-CHECK EVERY 8–12 WEEKS

② SUPPLEMENTS

DR. DALE'S

Cholest

DOSE 3 capsules in the PM for 6 weeks, then re-test.

DR. DALE'S

Bio Film Detox

DOSE 1 capsule twice daily, away from / between meals.

Biofilms are structured colonies of bacteria, fungi, or other microbes embedded in a protective matrix of polysaccharides and proteins. They adhere to surfaces — including the gut lining, oral cavity, sinuses, arterial plaques, and even medical implants — and this matrix makes them resistant to the immune system and to antimicrobial treatments.

DR. DALE'S

Hepatic Glutathione Pathway

> **DOSE** 3 capsules with the first meal of the day.

Opening the hepatic glutathione pathway can support a reduction in liver-driven inflammation and improve bile flow, which directly lowers cholesterol. It may reduce LDL oxidation (which drives plaque) and may decrease liver fat accumulation.

DR. DALE'S

Raw Nattokinase

> **DOSE** 2 capsules between meals, once or twice daily.

Nattokinase is a fibrinolytic enzyme extracted from natto, a traditional Japanese fermented soybean food made with *Bacillus subtilis natto*. It naturally breaks down fibrin — a protein involved in blood clot formation, and also a structural component of biofilms and microvascular inflammation. It acts as a systemic enzyme, working throughout the bloodstream rather than just in the digestive tract.

PURE ENCAPSULATIONS

CoQ10 — 250 mg

> **DOSE** 1 capsule twice daily with meals.

Supports both mitochondrial energy production and cardiovascular inflammation control — two areas often strained when cholesterol is elevated. CoQ10 specifically supports the liver's ability to process fat efficiently.

NORDIC NATURALS

Algae Omegas

> **DOSE** 2 gelcaps daily with a meal.

Directly reduce vascular inflammation and help correct the underlying lipid imbalance that drives cholesterol issues.

PURE ENCAPSULATIONS

Quercetin

> **DOSE** 2 capsules twice daily with meals.

Quercetin reduces oxidative stress, stabilizes blood vessels, prevents LDL oxidation, lowers inflammatory cytokines, and improves vascular function — making it a powerful adjunct when both cholesterol and inflammatory markers are elevated.

PURE ENCAPSULATIONS

L-Arginine

> **DOSE** 2 capsules 3× daily, taken on an empty stomach.

Directly supports nitric oxide production, which is essential for healthy blood vessel function.

RE-SYNC RECOVERY

Nitric Oxide Blend

> **DOSE** 1 scoop daily in cold or hot water. Ideal times: 1 hour before or after a workout, or 1 hour before bed.

QUICKSILVER SCIENTIFIC

Methylated B Complex — Lemon & Raspberry

> **DOSE** 2 pumps, hold for 30 seconds in the mouth, then swallow. Best taken with breakfast or shortly after waking.

Improves methylation, liver detoxification, homocysteine metabolism, and cardiovascular endothelial repair. This blend provides the proper activated forms of B vitamins, all required for proper methylation. When methylation is sluggish, the body builds up homocysteine — a major inflammatory molecule that damages blood vessels and increases LDL oxidation.

This protocol is provided for educational purposes and is intended for patients under the care of a qualified practitioner. It is not a substitute for individualized medical advice, diagnosis, or treatment. Functional ranges differ from standard lab reference ranges. Do not begin, stop, or adjust any supplement or medication — including cholesterol or blood-thinning medications — without consulting your provider, particularly if you are taking anticoagulants or managing a medical condition.

Chapter 3:
Stress & Energy Levels

You may be familiar with the terms "chronic fatigue", "adrenal insufficiency" and "adrenal burnout". The adrenals are two glands - one sitting on top of each kidney, that act as the body's stress-response command center. They produce hormones that help you adapt to physical, emotional, and environmental stressors. They not only regulate energy but also inflammation, blood sugar, blood pressure, electrolytes, and the body's overall resilience to stress.

The adrenals are responsible for:

- Keeping your energy stable throughout the day.
- Regulating your sleep-wake cycle.
- Managing inflammation.
- Controlling blood sugar and cravings.
- Helping maintain electrolyte and fluid balance.
- Influencing mood, resilience and stress tolerance.
- Supporting immune system balance.
- Contributing to sex hormone production - especially DHEA

Being that DHEA is the precursor to all hormones, it is imperative to have healthy adrenal glands if you want to have healthy sex hormone levels of testosterone, estrogen(s) and progesterone. The adrenals are also responsible for kicking into gear when the body goes into "fight or flight". Here is a very detailed example of the body's flight or fight response. Let's pretend that you are in the woods, and you see a bear:

1. First, the sympathetic nervous system prepares the body for action by increasing your heart rate - meaning your blood pressure goes up.

2. Your adrenals release the hormone adrenalin so that you have the energy to run. There is no possible way you can rest or sleep properly with this hormone coursing through your veins - it's time to run, not rest.

3. Blood sugar is also released into the blood stream - giving you energy to run. Meaning you temporarily have a rise in glucose levels.

4. Focus is also enhanced and the body diverts blood flow to muscles.

Unfortunately, in the modern world the stress that we are constantly under puts our Autonomic Nervous System in a chronic state of *"fight or flight."* Meaning our adrenals get stuck in that stress response mode. Looking at everything that happens to the body going into fight or flight, you can see how these become chronic issues with blood sugar, blood pressure, sleep and adrenal fluctuations if the body consistently thinks it is in fight or flight. This is why stress is so depleting and wreaks havoc on the body. We are not meant to be in a constant state of fight or flight.

Looking at the adrenals using saliva lab tests, you can see the cascade of adrenal hormones throughout the day. If cortisol production/release is low at any point, they are underperforming and if it is high they are in overdrive. Much like any other glands in the endocrine system, something can only overwork for so long before it burns out and goes into under-functioning.

Unfortunately, the American people along with most of the world are also severely addicted to caffeine and sugar. These stimulants place additional demands on your adrenals by putting them on a roller coaster all day. Caffeine is simply a plant-based pesticide chemical and once you come down, your adrenals attempt to stop your body from feeling the "crash". If you do not view sugar and caffeine as addictive chemicals that are bad for your health, I invite you to start looking at them as such substances. When your adrenals are "low" all day long - you're probably going to be tired. And if they are high - you may be too wired. I outline protocols to help with both scenarios. This may explain why you are tired in the morning but wired at night for example.

What if your tests come back and your adrenals are not the issue? The next step is to look at what is called the Krebs cycle and ATP production. The Krebs cycle (also called the citric acid cycle or TCA cycle) is a central metabolic pathway inside the mitochondria that turns the food you eat (carbs, proteins, and fats) into usable cellular energy in the form of ATP (adenosine triphosphate). This is the core engine of human energy production and when it slows down, energy levels can drop system wide.

The Krebs cycle involves a series of enzymatic reactions inside the mitochondria that take broken nutrients (known as acetyl-CoA), strip them of electrons and feed those electrons into the electron transport chains. ATP is produced from this process and is the molecule that your cells use for energy - I like to say it's the fuel that the cell combusts for energy. For this to happen properly, certain essential nutrients are key, especially B vitamins (B1, B2, B3 & B5), magnesium, lipoic acid, and CoQ10.

If you are dealing with energy issues, it is important to look at the Krebs cycle as well - not just the adrenals. You can evaluate how well your Krebs cycle is functioning using an organic acid test (OAT) as well as certain metabolic markers that assess each step of the cycle and how efficiently you're producing ATP. Also keep in mind if you have any of the symptoms listed above under being stuck in fight or flight, your nervous system may be stuck causing issues that relate to more than just your adrenals. It is important to properly evaluate to know what the cause of your fatigue is. It may be adrenals, ATP cycle, or potentially both.

The Organic Acid Test I recommend is from Mosaic Diagnostics and is one of the most effective ways to determine whether low energy is coming from a problem in the Krebs cycle, from mitochondrial function, or ATP production. It does this by measuring the metabolic by-products (organic acids) that your body produces when running the Krebs cycle and generating ATP. When these metabolites are too high or too low, it reveals exactly where the energy-production pathway is breaking down.

Here's how the test helps you evaluate whether low energy is caused by mitochondrial or ATP issues:

1. It Measures Each Step of the Krebs Cycle (TCA Cycle)

The OAT reports include markers such as:

- Citrate
- Isocitrate
- α-Ketoglutarate
- Succinate
- Fumarate
- Malate

When these are elevated, it means that step of the Krebs cycle is backed up, slowing ATP production. When they're low, it may indicate nutrient deficiency or poor mitochondrial turnover. This allows you to see *where* the energy block is occurring.

There is another major cause of low energy that is often overlooked and that is fatigue related to low hormones. Taking a saliva hormone test along with the other tests recommended will help you to determine the source(s) of your energy issues. Once a woman goes into perimenopause, sex hormones drop significantly. The caveat is, you may be in perimenopause and not know it if you are still having normal menstrual cycles every 28-ish days. Perimenopause is determined by hormone levels dropping rather than by a change in your cycle. If you have PCOS, this may happen years before your cycles change and you enter menopauses. This is why continuing to test and understand hormone levels consistently is important. If you have fatigue and determine that you have low hormone levels, this is an important avenue to explore.

As a naturopath who uses homeopathy, I want to mention that not everyone always responds to homeopathy. It is important to try the natural solutions first and to know that there is a backup net to catch you if all else fails. Homeopathy is great to balance the system and encourages native hormone production - it is also great to reduce menopause symptoms. But if you are looking to significantly raise hormone levels, or suffering from severe hormone-related fatigue, then HRT (Hormone Replacement Therapy) may become a viable option for you.

Should you either need or choose to use HRT, there are some important things that I would like you to understand. The first being, please monitor yourself often and use saliva testing rather than blood. I have seen hundreds of saliva hormone tests on women and men taking HRT that show certain hormones are way too high. When this happens, the hormone levels become toxic and dangerous. This needs to be avoided at all costs. Shockingly, many of my clients have reported to me that their hormone clinic physicians will only hormone test them every 2 years while using HRT. This is unacceptable and very lazy of clinicians. When using HRT, especially at the onset, more testing is not only necessary but required. Additionally, homeopathy can be used to help harmonize the HRT which can be hard to get balanced. I am providing a protocol for a combination of HRT and homeopathy for hormone "building".

I have designed this as one protocol, for which you will use what applies to you based on your labs. Because fatigue can have roots in several different areas, it will be your job to properly test all areas to rule out and confirm the singular or various root causes of your fatigue. Please do not do any sort of detoxification if you have extreme fatigue as it will further deplete you.

CLINICAL PROTOCOL · 100% NATURAL

Fatigue / Low Energy

Adrenal, mitochondrial & energy support

BY **DIANA M. DRAKE, BCTN** · DMD NATURAL MEDICINE

This protocol is designed for overall adrenal support, with targeted therapies for the specific cortisol times that test low or high. Remember: even if something is "in range," if it is skewing low or high, that matters — it's worth starting to balance from a preventative perspective.

① RECOMMENDED LABS

RUN ALL TO FIND THE ROOT CAUSE

ACCESS MEDICAL LABS

OpenDx Supreme Saliva Hormone Test

BLOOD PANEL

Iron, B12 & Copper

FUNCTIONAL TESTING

OAT — Organic Acid Test

ZRT LABORATORY

Thyroid Toxicity Panel

If the thyroid is underactive, run the **Thyroid** protocol as an adjunct to this one.

② CAFFEINE WEAN-OFF SCHEDULE

If you have fatigue, it is imperative that caffeine come out of your life as the energetic crutch it has become. Over time, your body's energy will come back and you will not need it. If you consume several caffeinated drinks daily, stretch this over 2 full months. The schedule below assumes coffee.

WEEK	REGIMEN
WEEK 1	75% regular · 25% decaf
WEEK 2	50% regular · 50% decaf
WEEK 3	75% decaf · 25% regular
WEEK 4	Stop — or, every other day, a small cup of green tea
WEEK 5	**STOP**

③ SUPPLEMENTS

DR. DALE'S

Adaptogen Pro

> DOSE 1–2 caps with the meals closest to the cortisol times that are out of balance.

DR. DALE'S

ATP Max

> DOSE 1–2 caps in the AM and again mid-morning or mid-afternoon, for cellular energy.

BIOTICS RESEARCH

Fe-Zyme (IF IRON IS LOW)

> DOSE 1 tablet daily in the AM.

Iron is imperative for energy, especially in women due to blood loss during the menstrual cycle. It supports proper energy levels, particularly if you know you are deficient. **Do not take iron if you have been tested and told you are high in iron.**

DR. DALE'S

Nano-Ionic Iodine

> DOSE 30 drops daily in water.

Proper iodine levels support thyroid function, which regulates cellular energy production.

> If deficient, or if you have never supplemented with iodine before, start with a loading dose of 90 drops daily, or try Dr. Dale's **Bio-Iodine** capsules (a much higher dose).

APEX ENERGETICS · TOPICAL ADRENAL CREAM

AdrenaStim or AdrenaCalm

> USE **AdrenaStim** for low cortisol · **AdrenaCalm** for high cortisol.
> Apply to the lower back (right onto the adrenals) during the times cortisol tested low or high. You can also apply to the inner arm, or alternate locations.

The adaptogenic herbs in these formulas are designed to support an increase or decrease of cortisol production in fatigued adrenal glands.

INJECTABLE COENZYME

NAD+ — 500 mg

> DOSE Reconstitute the bottle to the top of the neck with bacteriostatic water. 100–200 units, twice weekly for 2–4 weeks, then drop down to a maintenance dose.

Though NAD+ does not directly increase cortisol, it can help with the low energy associated with this condition. NAD+ also works on ATP and mitochondrial health, so it is a must-have if you have confirmed issues with your ATP production / Krebs cycle.

PURE ENCAPSULATIONS

DHEA — 5 mg (IF DHEA IS LOW)

> DOSE 1–3 caps in the AM daily.

DHEA is an adrenal hormone.

> It may be appropriate to add **pregnenolone** (another precursor) if DHEA and sex hormones are low. Ideally, try DHEA and/or pregnenolone **first** to see if they convert to the other hormones before adding estrogen, progesterone, or testosterone. You may only need one or the other — this is why it is so important to test often and understand how the hormones are working in your body.

④ MITOCHONDRIAL REPAIR — ATP / KREBS CYCLE

IF THE OAT TEST CONFIRMS MITOCHONDRIAL DYSFUNCTION

Morning Supplemental Stack

CoQ10	100–200 mg
Magnesium Citrate / Malate	200 mg
B Complex	1 capsule
Life Extension PQQ (Pyrroloquinoline Quinone)	10–20 mg
Nordic Naturals Algae Omega	1,000–2,000 mg

> PQQ stimulates the production of new mitochondria.

This protocol is provided for educational purposes and is intended for patients under the care of a qualified practitioner. It is not a substitute for individualized medical advice, diagnosis, or treatment. Run the recommended tests to identify or rule out root causes. Do not take iron unless testing confirms you are low. Do not begin, stop, or adjust any hormone, precursor, injectable, or supplement without consulting your provider, particularly if you are managing a medical condition.

Chapter 4
Digestive & Gut healing

The amount of information we now have about our gut health and microbiomes could fill a never-ending number of books. I would like to make this easy by categorizing the most likely root causes of gut issues and how to balance the digestive system naturally. The first rule to healing your microbiome is that you make an agreement with yourself never to take an antibiotic. Unless you are suffering from gangrene and about to lose a leg in the hospital and it is a life-threatening emergency, an antibiotic is not appropriate for the other 99% of scenarios - even some emergency scenarios. Things like strep throat, sinus infections, bacterial vaginosis, kidney infections etc. are among the most common things that will have you on a hamster wheel of continuing to take antibiotics while wrecking your microbiome in the meantime.

If you experienced frequent childhood infections, you were likely prescribed multiple rounds of antibiotics. We now understand that this disrupts the gut microbiome and weakens immune function later in life. To understand why, we need to briefly explore terrain theory vs. germ theory.

The body's "Terrain" is the internal biological environment. This includes cellular heath, mineral balance, pH and acid-base balance, oxygen levels, mitochondrial function, microbiome composition, detoxification capacity, immune system function, inflammatory state, nutrient availability and hormone state. Terrain theory is the concept that disease develops naturally due to an unhealthy internal environment in the body rather than exposure to "catching germs". Western medicine has built their entire system on the opposite scientific theory called "Germ Theory". Germ theory is based on the supposition that disease is caused by an "invasion" of bad bacteria and viruses with specific strains causing specific diseases.

The genesis of these theories began in the 1850's between Louis Pasteur and Antoine Bechamp. You can read about this incredible turning point in history and see the research put forth by both parties in several modern books including, *Bechamp or Pasteur? A Lost Chapter in the History of Biology* by Ethel Douglas Hume. Much like the story of Nikola Tesla who was defunded, defamed and destroyed, you will find a similar history with Germ and Terrain theory. And in case you're wondering who won, it was the theory that makes the most profit. If you are afraid of "catching germs" and "getting sick from other people" then you will invest in sanitation, vaccines, antibiotics and the hysteria of fear that you are going to get or make another person sick.

You've probably heard the phrase, *"your immune system lives in your gut,"* but what does that mean? Think of your body as a sophisticated waste-management and recycling facility. Everything you interact with—air, water, sunlight, food—must be evaluated by the body and sorted. Each input becomes either something the body can use, or something the body must discard. Literally - trash or treasure. When you understand this simple principle, you gain a powerful framework for understanding your health. From a naturopathic perspective, disease arises from only two fundamental issues:

1. Deficiency — not enough of something the body requires.

2. Toxicity — too much of something the body cannot use or safely eliminate. This is called "toxemia".

Even many genetically inherited conditions ultimately trace back to a point in ancestry where DNA became damaged or altered—either through lack of essential nutrients or through toxic exposure that disrupted normal genetic expression.

When we talk about the immune system, what exactly are we referring to? It isn't a single organ you can point to… Instead, it functions as the body's trash and removal network. Its job is simple yet vital: to distinguish *"self"* from *"non-self"* and eliminate anything that does not belong. This system is made up of a variety of bacteria that help break down and "consume" waste, as well as the lymphatic vessels, fluid, and nodes that transport and remove that waste. Supporting this filtration process are the skin, liver, kidneys, and colon—all of which serve as major routes of elimination.

Your entire body is constantly working to process and expel metabolic byproducts, toxins, and environmental chemicals. And in today's world, this system is continually overburdened. Our modern environment exposes us to far more toxins than the body was designed to handle, a concept we will explore more deeply in the chapter on detoxification.

Your microbiome is a vast network of microorganisms that outnumber your human cells—an extraordinary thought. These microbes form an ecosystem that supports digestion, immunity, hormone balance, detoxification, and communication throughout the body. Contrary to the idea that "bad bacteria" are only acquired from the outside world, many organisms—*including various strains of streptococcus*—are normal, resident members of the human microbiome. They live in balance with the rest of your microbial community. Problems arise not simply because these bacteria appear, but because the internal terrain becomes imbalanced, creating a demand for the more aggressive bacteria to grow. For example, rather than looking at strep throat as an infection that you "caught", consider the possibility that it may be caused by inflammation due to toxicity and poor lymphatic flow in the tonsils and throat area. This toxemia of the throat causes your body to signal the immune system to make more strep bacteria in this area to clean up the garbage. The reason strep often returns after a round of antibiotics is because all you really did was kill the garbage men, but the trash is still there and needs to be removed.

When the body is under stress, toxic burden increases, tissues become congested, or immunity becomes compromised and these normally quiet microbes will multiply, on purpose, because there is a demand for them. In many naturopathic models, this is understood as the body attempting to break down damaged tissue, congestion, or metabolic waste that it cannot clear on its own.

To illustrate the relationship between terrain, stagnation, and microbial shifts, I'll share an example from my own clinical journey. Several years ago, I underwent a holistic dental procedure to clean old extraction sites where my wisdom teeth had been removed fifteen years earlier by a conventional dentist. When teeth are removed conventionally, the bone sometimes fails to heal properly, forming what is known as a *cavitation*—a small area of unhealed bone that can accumulate stagnant blood and tissue.

When these cavitations were opened and cleaned, the samples sent to the lab showed the presence of streptococcal species and other bacteria. This didn't mean I had an active strep throat infection. In fact, I had never had strep throat in my life. Instead, these organisms were growing in an enclosed space where blood flow was poor, tissue breakdown was occurring, and the body needed microbial assistance to manage stagnation. In other words, the environment in that pocket needed the strep bacteria to work on breaking down all the garbage that was caught in those closed sockets.

Recurring sinus or ear infections are not simply the result of "catching bad bacteria" from an airplane, a classroom, or a crowded environment. These conditions more often reflect an internal terrain problem buildup of congestion, stagnation, and cellular debris in the very pathways the body uses for elimination and drainage. When these tissues become overburdened, the microbiome shifts. Certain bacteria multiply to break down accumulated waste inflammation increases, and symptoms appear. In this view, the infection is not the cause of the problem, but a response to imbalance. In other words - the infection is the result of the poor terrain.

Viruses also behave differently than the popular narrative suggests. Rather than being free-living organisms that survive independently in nature, viruses are cell-dependent particles that only replicate inside living cells. Viruses cannot be grown on their own in isolation the way bacteria can— viruses require host tissue to replicate. From a terrain perspective, viral activity reflects the state of the host: the level of toxicity, stress, immune burden, nutrient deficiency, and environmental overwhelm. The question becomes less *"What did I catch?"* and more *"What is my body trying to detox?"*

This is why, in the same household or on the same plane, some individuals get sick while others remain completely unaffected. The difference lies not solely in exposure, but in resilience, detoxification capacity, and the condition of the internal terrain. On a plane, you are being exposed to electromagnetic fields (AKA radiation), jet fuel fumes, dehydration, likely improper nutrition, and the stress of travel.

Fear itself is often the most contagious element during outbreaks. When we instead understand symptoms as the body's effort to rebalance and clear what it no longer needs, we can approach illness with far more clarity and far less fear.

The microorganisms that live within your body play an essential role in maintaining balance, breaking down waste, and supporting health. After death, these same microbes continue their natural process of decomposition — not because they are "attacking" the body, but because their role is to break down tissue, both in life and afterward. In that sense, bacteria function more as decomposers and recyclers than fighters.

Your gut is home to trillions of these organisms. The kinds of foods, chemicals, and environmental exposures you encounter in shape which microbes thrive. When you nourish your body with healthy, whole foods, your microbiome develops communities of bacteria that support digestion, immunity, and overall wellness. When your system is exposed to more processed foods, chemicals, or irritants, the microbial balance shifts toward species that are better suited to break down those substances. In other words, your microbiome adapts to *what you feed it and what your body needs to help processing.* The microbial environment you carry reflects your internal terrain.

This concept lies at the heart of terrain theory: the idea that health or illness depends more on the condition of the internal environment than on external "germs." If you're interested in diving deeper into this perspective, I highly recommend exploring the following books:

1. *Goodbye Germ Theory* by Author, **Dr. William Trebing**

2. *AIDS, Opium, Diamonds, and Empire: The Deadly Virus of International Greed* by Author, **Nancy Turner Banks**

3. *What Really Makes You Ill? Why Everything You Thought You Knew About Disease Is Wrong* , written by authors, **Dawn Lester and David Parker**.

Imagine your body as a **pond.** If the water is not filtered properly, various organisms can begin to grow—scum, algae, mold, and bacteria. The pond doesn't become overrun because something "attacked" it from the outside; it becomes overrun because the environment inside it changed. It became stagnant, congested, and overburdened. Your body works the same way.

Your liver, kidneys, colon, lymphatic system, and skin function as your natural filtration and elimination systems. They are designed to remove metabolic waste, environmental toxins, and byproducts of normal cellular activity. But in today's world—filled with chemical exposures, processed foods, chronic stress, and environmental pollutants, these systems can become *severely* overburdened. And this concept of toxemia isn't even acknowledged by Western Medical

Doctors. When your body's filters cannot keep up, internal stagnation develops, creating a terrain where unwanted symptoms, inflammation, and microbial imbalance can thrive.

Think of it this way:

1. **The pond must be filtered.**
   This represents the body's own detox organs doing their job.

2. **The filter must be cleaned via maintenance.**
   This represents intentional detoxification practices that support and reset those organs when they become overburdened.

Both steps are necessary for a healthy environment, both in a pond and your very own body. I go into much more detail on this process—and how to support each detoxification pathway—in the dedicated chapter on detoxification.

To get to the bottom of your gut issues there are a lot of different tests you can take. If you have severe issues, I recommend you take all these tests at some point. In order of importance:

1. Food Sensitivity Testing

Understanding whether a particular food is triggering inflammation in your gut is essential for healing. When a food sensitivity panel comes back with a long list of reactive foods, it often indicates that your gut lining is compromised and the immune system is overactive. In these cases, the issue is rarely the food itself but points to an inflamed state of your gut. During healing, these reactive foods should be removed to give the digestive and immune systems a chance to calm down. After 90 days to 6 months on one of my gut-repair protocols, foods can be reintroduced slowly, one at a time, to evaluate your tolerance.

Please be aware that food "sensitivities" (referred to as IgG) are different than "allergies" (referred to as IgE). True IgE-mediated allergies are different from sensitivities and must be avoided indefinitely. Celiac disease, for example, is an autoimmune condition in which gluten exposure creates significant immune activation and intestinal damage. It's important to acknowledge here the impact of modern agricultural practices on how the body responds to wheat. Wheat grown and processed in the United States has undergone extensive hybridization (this means it is genetically modified) over time and is commonly treated with chemicals during harvesting and processing. Domestic wheat is sprayed with toxic glyphosate (Round Up) chemicals during the harvesting process. It is then bleached and bromine is added - another toxic chemical causing an array of health issues. I will speak more on issues with bromine in my thyroid chapter. Many of my clients report that they tolerate breads, pasta, and other wheat-based foods more easily while eating and traveling abroad. In many regions outside the U.S., wheat is grown differently, minimally processed, and prepared using traditional methods such as sourdough fermentation, which can improve digestibility.

For those who choose to consume wheat, organic and traditionally prepared varieties are often better tolerated and less likely to provoke an inflammatory response.

2. Gut Barrier Function + Candida (checking for leaky gut & candida)

This panel evaluates markers of increased intestinal permeability, commonly referred to as "leaky gut." In this condition, the tight junctions of the gut lining become compromised, allowing partially digested food particles, endotoxins, and microbial byproducts to move into your bloodstream or lymphatic system. When this happens, your immune system flags these substances as foreign and initiates an inflammatory response to remove them.

Because your lymphatic system drains toward the skin— your largest elimination organ—these internal reactions can sometimes manifest externally as rashes, eczema, acne, hives, or other negative skin conditions. In naturopathic medicine, skin symptoms are viewed as a reflection of what is happening internally at the gut and immune level.

This panel also tests for candida overgrowth. Candida is a naturally occurring yeast that is part of a healthy digestive ecosystem. However, when beneficial bacteria are depleted—often due to stress, antibiotic use, poor diets, or immune imbalance—candida can increase beyond normal levels. Excessive sugar and refined carbohydrates further fuel this overgrowth, which can contribute to bloating, fatigue, cravings, inflammation, and recurrent infections.

Understanding both intestinal permeability and candida balance is a crucial step toward identifying what is driving inflammation in the body and creating a targeted plan for gut healing.

3. G.I. Map

G.I. mapping tests can be incredibly informative, but they also tend to be more expensive and come in many different formats. If you decide to go this route, I highly recommend working with a practitioner who specializes in gut health. They can help you interpret the results accurately and guide you toward the right probiotics and targeted supplements to rebalance your microbiome. Additionally, there are a lot of companies that offer some great at home test kits and include not only user-friendly reports - but supplemental recommendations as well. Viome is an example of that although their test does not include a parasite panel which I feel is important. Keep in mind - a negative on a parasite panel may not necessarily mean you don't have them. They tend to nest and hide very well in the gut lining. This is why parasite cleansing is important to do twice yearly, and I will cover that in my detoxification chapter. Parasite cleansing is also included in my master gut reboot protocol for this chapter as well.

If you're choosing a G.I. test on your own, look for one that evaluates not only your microbial balance but also screens for **parasites, molds, and yeast.** Some tests even include **food sensitivity markers** based on stool analysis, allowing you to gather multiple insights in one panel. There are now even **genetic tests** focused specifically on gut function—so the options truly are endless. Rather than listing every test available, my lab shops feature a handful of good options to choose from if you do not want to source something from the internet.

CLINICAL PROTOCOL · 100% NATURAL

Total Digestive Rejuvenation

A three-phase gut reset: Remove · Repopulate · Rebuild

BY **DIANA M. DRAKE, BCTN** · DMD NATURAL MEDICINE

PHASE 1	PHASE 2	PHASE 3
Remove	**Repopulate**	**Rebuild the Lining**
8–12 weeks	6–8 weeks	—

RECOMMENDED LABS

ALLETESS MEDICAL LABS

IgG Food Sensitivity Testing

US BIOTEK

GI Basic Profile Map — with bacteria, yeast & parasite profile

QUEST DIAGNOSTICS

H. Pylori Breath Test

> Add the H. Pylori test if you have skin conditions such as rosacea; burning or gnawing stomach pain in the upper abdomen; pain when the stomach is empty (between meals or at night); bloating; frequent burping; nausea; loss of appetite; or unintentional weight loss. If these symptoms don't sound like you, you can skip it.

① PHASE 1 — REMOVE 8–12 WEEKS

The amount of time on this phase should reflect the severity of the symptoms and imbalances on your test results.

DR. DALE'S

Bio-Tox Total Bacteria

DOSE 5 droppers full daily.

Use this remedy to reduce any overgrown bacterial strains.

DR. DALE'S

BioTox Total Fungus

DOSE 5 droppers full daily.

Use this remedy if yeast, molds, or candida are found in the system. You will also want to adopt an anti-fungal diet during this time (see the Candida Control Diet below).

CANDIDA CONTROL DIET

✓ YOU CAN EAT

PROTEIN
Meat, eggs, protein powder. Always organic.

COMPLEX CARBOHYDRATES
Non-starchy veggies — all greens, tomatoes, peppers, etc.

FRUIT
Frozen berries (freezing removes the mold), lemons, grapefruit. No other fruit.

BEANS
Black & pinto. Chili is a great meal.

GRAINS
Old-fashioned oatmeal is the ONLY grain you can have.

FATS
Olive oil, coconut, almonds, peanut butter (stir in a little colloidal silver to kill mold). If you want cheese, eat goat cheese.

✗ YOU CANNOT EAT

- No starchy foods: potatoes, carrots, rice, wheat, grains (except old-fashioned oatmeal), bread, pasta, cake, pizza, etc.
- No cheese, milk, cream, or dairy; no vinegar, mushrooms, mayo, or mustard.
- Absolutely no sugar: no soda, cookies, sweets, candy, honey, agave, maple syrup, etc.
- No high-sugar fruits: bananas, mangos, kiwi, apples, pineapple, oranges, pears, peaches, etc. Only the fruits listed at left.
- No juices, especially store-bought. Fresh-pressed is OK only if it is green juice free of the sweet/sugary fruits.

> Candida thrives on sugar — or anything that turns into sugar. The object of this diet is to starve the yeast so it has nothing to eat and begins to die off. Cheating in any way will prolong your symptoms.

DR. DALE'S

Bio Film Detox

> **DOSE** 1 capsule 15 minutes before meals.

Helps break down biofilms.

DR. DALE'S · LIQUID

Bio Tox Total Parasite

> **DOSE** 5 droppers full once daily.

DR. DALE'S

Para-Pro

> **DOSE** 2 capsules per meal with food.

Regardless of whether you tested positive for parasites, it is a good idea to run a parasite cleanse while you are trying to reset the gut.

DR. DALE'S

Colon Pro

> **DOSE** 1–2 capsules with every meal. Take enough to move the colon; if diarrhea occurs, reduce the dose by 1 capsule.

Colon Pro acts as a binder and colon detoxification formula.

MICROBIOME LABS

Pylo Guard (IF PYLORI IS POSITIVE)

> **DOSE** 1 capsule daily.

② PHASE 2 — REPOPULATE 6–8 WEEKS

DR. DALE'S

Microbiome Terrain Pro

DOSE 1 capsule with each meal.

Repopulates good bacteria with spore-forming probiotics and works on gut-lining integrity and repair.

DR. DALE'S

Digest Pro

DOSE 2 capsules in the AM & PM, and before every meal.

Helps repair digestive processes by encouraging native production of enzymes and stomach acid. Contains no microbes.

Customized Probiotic Stack

Based on the good strains that were **low** on your test, find supplements that contain those specific strains. You may need several different products to replace everything you need.

> A quick way to build the list: enter the strains you were low on into an AI assistant (such as ChatGPT) and ask for product recommendations that contain them.

③ PHASE 3 — REBUILD THE GUT LINING

This phase rebuilds and heals the gut lining after the terrain has been cleared and repopulated.

MICROBIOME LABS

MegaMucosa — capsules or powder

DOSE Take as directed.

INTEGRATIVE THERAPEUTICS

Gut Healing Powder

DOSE Take as directed.

DR. DALE'S

Bio Age Reverse — Vitamin C & Collagen Powder

DOSE 1 scoop 3× daily in a short glass with juice, or in a smoothie.

DR. DALE'S

Digest Pro

DOSE 2 capsules in the AM & PM, and before every meal.

Continue Digest Pro through Phases 2 and 3 to keep supporting enzyme and stomach-acid production. Contains no microbes.

Take all as directed *to rebuild and reseal the gut lining.*

CLINICAL PROTOCOL · 100% NATURAL

Lack of Bowel Movements / Colon Congestion

Colon detoxification & regularity support

BY **DIANA M. DRAKE, BCTN** · DMD NATURAL MEDICINE

① SUPPLEMENTS

DR. DALE'S

Colon Pro

> DOSE 1–2 capsules with every meal. Take enough to move the colon; if diarrhea occurs, reduce the dose by 1 capsule.

Colon Pro acts as a binder and colon detoxification formula.

DR. DALE'S

Nano-Ionic Multi-Mineral with Silica

> DOSE Add 30 drops to every 20 oz serving of water.

ANY BRAND

Magnesium Oxide

> DOSE 300–500 mg at night.

Any brand is fine — look for a veggie capsule free of magnesium stearate.

DR. DALE'S

Microbiome Terrain Pro

> DOSE 1–2 capsules 3× daily with meals.

② DIETARY RECOMMENDATIONS

1. **Increase fiber-based foods** — fruits, veggies, and greens.
2. **Increase hydration** with well-mineralized water.

This protocol is provided for educational purposes and is intended for patients under the care of a qualified practitioner. It is not a substitute for individualized medical advice, diagnosis, or treatment. Persistent constipation, or a sudden change in bowel habits, should be evaluated by your provider. Do not begin, stop, or adjust any supplement without consulting your provider, particularly if you are pregnant, nursing, taking medications, or managing a medical condition.

CLINICAL PROTOCOL · 100% NATURAL

Acid Indigestion

Acid backing up into the esophagus — with potential nausea & vomiting

BY **DIANA M. DRAKE, BCTN** · DMD NATURAL MEDICINE

① RECOMMENDED LABS

QUEST DIAGNOSTICS

H. Pylori Breath Test

WHY THIS MATTERS

The presence of H. Pylori in the gut is typically the result of **low stomach acid** from a poor diet high in overly acidic foods. That same low stomach acid is what causes acid reflux — food sits in the stomach too long, begins to ferment, and bubbles back up. Note the add-on supplement below that is needed **only if H. Pylori is present.** If you test positive for H. Pylori, also run the full **Total Digestive Rejuvenation** protocol along with Pylo Guard.

② SUPPLEMENTS

DR. DALE'S

Digest Pro

DOSE 2 caps in the AM, 2 caps with each meal, 2 caps in the PM.

Supports restoration of native digestive function and acid production.

Heartburn Relief

DOSE 2 tablets after a meal that causes indigestion.

MICROBIOME LABS

Pylo Guard (IF PYLORI IS POSITIVE)

DOSE 1 capsule daily.

NATURAL FACTORS

Chewable Ginger

DOSE 1 before each meal.

③ DIETARY CHANGES — ELIMINATE

The goal is to stop the assault on the stomach from highly acidic foods. Eliminate the following:

1. ACID-SUPPRESSING & ACID-DILUTING

- Large volumes of liquid with meals
- Carbonated beverages
- Alcohol (especially wine, beer)
- Coffee
- Mint / peppermint
- Chocolate

2. HIGHLY FERMENTABLE CARBS (FODMAP-HEAVY)

These increase gas → push acid upward

- Wheat, rye, barley
- Onions, garlic (raw especially)
- Beans, lentils, chickpeas
- Apples, pears
- Honey, agave, HFCS
- Cauliflower, cabbage, Brussels sprouts
- Dairy with lactose (milk, soft cheeses)

3. REFINED & PROCESSED

- White sugar
- Pastry, crackers, cereals
- Ultra-processed snack foods
- Artificial sweeteners (sucralose, sorbitol)

4. INFLAMMATORY FATS

- Fried foods
- Seed oils (corn, soybean, canola)
- Heavy cream sauces

5. SPICY FOODS

- Hot peppers
- Wasabi
- Horseradish
- Hot sauces

This protocol is provided for educational purposes and is intended for patients under the care of a qualified practitioner. It is not a substitute for individualized medical advice, diagnosis, or treatment. Persistent reflux, difficulty swallowing, vomiting, or unintentional weight loss should be evaluated by your provider. Do not begin, stop, or adjust any supplement without consulting your provider, particularly if you are pregnant, nursing, taking medications, or managing a medical condition.

CLINICAL PROTOCOL · 100% NATURAL

Stomach Acid Rebuilding

Hydrochloric acid (HCl) titration

BY **DIANA M. DRAKE, BCTN** · DMD NATURAL MEDICINE

⚠ **Do not do this protocol if you have an active ulcer.**
You may need to have your upper digestive tract scoped by a medical doctor to find out whether it is an ulcer. Alternatively, you can try this protocol — but if, on the very first meal of taking an HCl supplement, you feel **pain**, please **DO NOT CONTINUE** this portion of the protocol.

① THE SUPPLEMENT & HOW TO BEGIN

PURE ENCAPSULATIONS

Betaine HCl Pepsin — 250 caps

PURPOSE: To restore adequate stomach acid levels and improve digestion.

- Use a hydrochloric acid (HCl) capsule (often combined with pepsin).
- Take capsules **immediately before meals** — never on an empty stomach.
- This protocol is intended for **meals that contain protein**.

② TITRATION SCHEDULE

MEAL	DAY 1	DAY 2
Before breakfast	1 capsule	4 capsules
Before lunch	2 capsules	5 capsules
Before dinner	3 capsules	6 capsules

Ongoing increase: continue increasing the dose by one additional capsule per meal each day, until you feel heartburn. Always take capsules right before eating, not on an empty stomach.

③ THE PROCESS

1 **WHAT TO WATCH FOR**

The key symptom to monitor is **heartburn, burning, or discomfort** in the chest or upper stomach. This sensation indicates you have reached more acid than your body currently needs.

2 **WHEN PAIN OCCURS**

- Stop increasing immediately.
- Reduce the dose by one capsule per meal.
- This reduced dose becomes your daily **maintenance dose**.

3 **MAINTENANCE PHASE**

Take the established dose before every meal, every day, and continue until it again causes discomfort. When discomfort returns, reduce the dose by one capsule and continue at the new lower dose. Keep repeating — each time a dose causes discomfort, drop by one capsule — so your dose steps down over time.

4 **COMPLETION OF THE PROTOCOL**

Over time, your required dose will naturally decrease. Many people eventually stabilize at 1–2 capsules before each meal, or none at all. When you no longer need supplemental HCl, your stomach acid levels are considered replenished and your digestion should be noticeably improved.

This protocol is provided for educational purposes and is intended for patients under the care of a qualified practitioner. It is not a substitute for individualized medical advice, diagnosis, or treatment. Do not perform HCl titration if you have an active ulcer, gastritis, or are taking NSAIDs, corticosteroids, or acid-blocking medications; stop immediately if you experience pain. When in doubt, have your upper digestive tract evaluated by a medical doctor. Do not begin, stop, or adjust any supplement without consulting your provider.

Chapter 5
Detoxification

We are being exposed to toxins from every possible angle. As mentioned in the last chapter, your body functions like a garbage-sorting facility. It has built-in filters designed to process waste—but when those filters are overwhelmed, problems begin at the cellular level. Think of it this way: imagine being handed a gallon of water and told, "There's poison in here, but it's diluted enough to be considered safe." Technically, your body can handle small amounts of toxins. What's never acknowledged is that these exposures don't happen in isolation. They happen all at once every day, from countless sources—and no one is calculating the combined load on the human body or the environment. For example, pregnant women are warned not to eat raw fish due to potential mercury poisoning, yet the combined metal load in early childhood vaccines exceeds what is considered safe for a 150-pound adult. The only real solution is personal responsibility:

- Active detoxification protocols
- Intentional nutrition
- Reducing exposure wherever possible

This exposure doesn't start in adulthood. It begins before you're even born. The first nine months of life are spent marinating in the toxic burden that your mother carries in her blood and amniotic fluid. What she eats, you eat. Whatever toxins are stored in her body, you are immersed in them for nearly a year. After birth, exposure often increases rather than decreases:

- Infants are injected with toxic vaccines.
- Breast milk can contain environmental toxins stored by the mother.
- Baby formulas may contain heavy metals, seed oils, and corn syrup.

Because of this, pregnancy pre-planning matters. Ideally, conception should be preceded by one to two years of intentional detoxification to reduce the toxic burden passed to the next generation.

More toxic exposure includes wearing synthetic clothing made from plastic from childhood to adulthood. Drinking from plastic bottles and playing with plastic toys - sucking on a plastic pacifier, eating from plastic containers and bags. Even baby mattresses and materials in the nursery are toxic unless intentionally selected and purchased from natural manufacturers. Even having vinyl flooring in your home off-gasses chemicals into your entire living space. Household products are highly toxic as well. Children have literally died or been hospitalized from accidentally eating laundry detergent pods. Yet instead of those companies making them non-toxic, they change the packaging to be "childproof". This is so backwards and yet people still invest in these chemicals. Most people are living inside a 360-degree dome of chemical exposure without realizing it. If you live in the United States, tap water is not fit for human consumption. Municipal tap water is heavily contaminated. Many contaminants are not routinely tested for, including:

- Glyphosate
- Microplastics
- Prescription drug residues

In addition, tap water commonly contains:

- **Fluoride,** a known neurotoxin.
- **Chlorine,** which disrupts stomach acid, gut flora, and the oral microbiome.
- **Heavy metals** often leak from aging pipes.

Water is foundational to every process in the body. When the foundation is contaminated, everything built on top of it suffers. Unfortunately, changing your drinking water is not enough. Bathing in city water causes these toxins to be absorbed through your skin and inhaled as vapors into your lungs. Environmental pollution is everywhere you turn. Pollution isn't limited to water. It's in:

- Our air
- Our oceans
- Our soil
- Our food supply
- Our homes

On top of chemical exposure, we are constantly bathing in electromagnetic radiation (referred to as EMFs) from:

- Cell towers
- Power lines
- Cell phones
- Wi-Fi routers
- Electrical wiring and appliances

These frequencies interact with metals in the body, essentially turning them into antennas. The result is radiation being redistributed throughout tissues. These frequencies have downstream effects, including:

- Drainage of ATP and mitochondrial energy production
- Altered water structure in the body, especially the blood
- Reduced oxygen delivery to cells due to blood cell clumping
- Impaired circulation and tissue health
- Disruption of the circadian rhythm causing poor sleep

Certain frequencies are particularly problematic and have been associated with lung tissue stress, compromised lung barrier function, and fluid accumulation. Your body runs on oxygen and energy. Anything that interferes with either will eventually show up as dysfunction.

Common Sources of Chemical Exposure

Some of the most frequent contributors include:

- Tap water
- Processed and packaged foods
- Synthetic clothing and fabrics
- Vinyl flooring and building materials
- Household cleaners and fragrances
- Personal care products
- Pesticides and herbicides (billions of these are dumped into the environment every single year)
- EMF exposure from modern technology

For the record, Vaccines contain the following:

1. Aluminum Salts
Forms: aluminum hydroxide, aluminum phosphate
Purpose: immune adjuvant (improves antibody response)

Concerns raised:

- Neurotoxicity at high doses
- Accumulation in kidney or neurologic disease

2. Thimerosal (Ethylmercury)
Purpose: preservative (prevents bacterial contamination in multi-dose vials)
Concerns raised:

- Mercury exposure
- Neurologic toxicity
- **Removed from nearly all childhood vaccines** in the U.S. however it is still used in **some multi-dose influenza vaccines**

3. Formaldehyde
Purpose: inactivates viruses and toxins during manufacturing
Concerns raised:

- Carcinogenicity at high or chronic exposures

4. Polysorbate 80

Purpose: emulsifier and stabilizer

Concerns raised:

- Increased gut permeability
- Possible allergic reactions

5. Residual Antibiotics

Examples: neomycin, polymyxin B, streptomycin

Purpose: prevent bacterial contamination during production

Concerns raised:

- Allergic reactions
- Microbiome effects

6. Egg Proteins

Purpose: residual from virus growth medium (e.g., influenza vaccines)

Concerns raised:

- Allergic reactions

7. Yeast Proteins

Purpose: by-product of recombinant manufacturing

Concerns raised:

- Allergic or immune reactions
- Potential to cause long term auto-immune issues

8. Gelatin

Purpose: stabilizer (prevents vaccine degradation)

Concerns raised:

- Allergic reactions
- Religious or dietary concerns

9. Residual Cell Culture Materials

Examples: fetal bovine serum, Vero cell proteins

Purpose: virus growth during manufacturing

Concerns raised:

- Immune sensitization

10. mRNA Vaccine Lipid Nanoparticles AKA "hydrogel"

Private research data on live blood analysis on vaccinated vs non-vaccinated individuals shows heavy burden of a new type of "nano-gel" that is behaving in an intelligent manner in the body.

Components: Unknown, new biotechnology

Purpose: Unknown and suspected sinister in nature. These hydrogels can replicate and potentially broadcast and receive signals, data and instruction to and from your body.

Plastics & Food Packaging Chemicals

Primary risk: Endocrine disruption, fertility issues, cancer risk

- **Bisphenols** (BPA, BPS, BPF)
- **Phthalates** (DEHP, DBP, DEP)
- **PFAS** ("forever chemicals" – PFOA, PFOS)
- **Styrene** (foam containers, polystyrene)
- **Vinyl chloride** (PVC plastics)

Common sources include:

Plastic food containers, water bottles, can linings, receipts, food wrap

2. Personal Care & Cosmetics

- **Primary risk:** Hormone disruption, neurotoxicity, immune effects
- **Parabens** (methyl-, propyl-, butyl-)
- **Synthetic fragrances** ("fragrance/parfum")
- **Triclosan**
- **Formaldehyde & formaldehyde releasers**
- **Oxybenzone & octinoxate** (chemical sunscreens)
- **Coal tar dyes**
- **Heavy metals** (lead in lipstick, arsenic in pigments

3. Household Cleaners & Indoor Air

Primary risk: Respiratory damage, hormone interference, neurological effects

- **Ammonia**
- **Chlorine & chloramines**
- **Quaternary ammonium compounds (quats)**
- **Volatile Organic Compounds** (VOCs) (benzene, toluene, xylene, formaldehyde)
- **Glycol ethers**

Sources:

Sprays, disinfectants, air fresheners, scented candles, dryer sheets, dish soap, dish washer soap and laundry detergent. Note that detergents labeled "free and clear" are simply free of perfumes and dyes but are still laden with toxins and chemical surfactants.

4. Geo-Engineering (Chemtrails)

Do not be fooled by claims that spraying our skies is a conspiracy. You need only to put your phone down and look up into your sky. The claims that these are "water vapor" trails that magically fog out and block the sun - that were never there until the early 2000's - are a lie. Several states have passed legislation to ban the spraying of the skies (aka Geoengineering). However, as this happens at the federal level, the handful of states that have done this are powerless and still experience this chemical fog. The toxins being sprayed into our atmosphere not only fall to the ground and into our water but also affect plant and animal life. Private researchers are testing rainwater, snow, human and animal blood. Their findings include a surge in the following metals and the addition of nano-bot technology in nature and living creatures including humans:

1. **Sulfur Dioxide (SO_2)**
2. **Calcium Carbonate ($CaCO_3$)**
3. **Aluminum Oxide (Al_2O_3)**
4. **Diamond Dust / Titanium Dioxide**
5. **Nanotechnology (small, parasite-like technology)**

Private research studying the environmental impact of chem-trails through the analysis of snow fall, rainwater and human tissue are reporting an "unknown" hybrid technology that appears to be a type of mechanism that interacts with the body. Nano-bots are envisioned as tiny machines that could:

- Move through fluids (like blood)
- Sense of their environment
- Perform specific tasks
- Respond to chemical or electromagnetic signals
- Replicate themselves
- Me be undetectable to the immune system and therefore will not be flagged to remove
- May severely flag the immune response in sensitive individuals causing a complete collapse in health and quality of life while going undiagnosed.

Now that you are armed with this information, it is essential to build detoxification protocols into your life every quarter, or at a minimum, every spring and fall. You are welcome to test your body for specific contaminants, and I will provide resources to help you do so. Please understand that specialized tests are expensive, and there is no single test that covers the full spectrum of every possible contaminant, all in one lab. Also, remember that toxins are stored in your body's tissues; they may not all show up properly on a test if they are stuck. Sometimes, multiple body fluid samples are needed to get a clear picture of the burden. For example, to assess heavy metals, it is ideal to analyze hair, blood, and urine rather than rely on a single sample type.

Most toxins in your body are the result of the toxic burden in the American environment. If you have specific symptoms, I recommend testing and doing target-specific detoxification. This scenario would 100% involve an array of tests to determine which toxin is most abundant and how best to remove it. For the most part, general detoxification targets the blood, lymphatic system, and organs to help rid the body of an array of overburdening chemicals via the proper elimination systems.

Please be aware of "The Detox Flu." When we begin to remove toxins from the cells and flush them out, they can make you feel sick. Headaches, fatigue, lethargy, vomiting, diarrhea, sweating, etc., are all possible if too many toxins come out too quickly. It is essential to understand that this is not something you "push through," but instead to back off on your detox remedies until the body returns to a normal state. Finding balance is the key - you want the toxins to come out slowly and safely. During detoxification protocols, drinking purified water with added minerals and electrolytes is incredibly important. The body cannot properly eliminate toxins when dehydrated, and drinking tap water during a detox is not recommended. Please do not ever drink tap water that comes from the city. It is ideal to follow a diet free of caffeine, sugar, animal products (including flesh and dairy), and gluten to help your body clear toxins during detoxification protocols.

Per terrain theory, when the junk builds up, the eater will come. I have included parasite detoxification in this section because it is important. We all have them. It is always possible to encounter more while traveling but not traveling doesn't make you exempt. Parasite cleansing needs to happen once or twice yearly especially if you:

- Have pets
- Travel
- Eat sushi (raw fish)
- Experience any kind of digestive issues

CLINICAL PROTOCOL · 100% NATURAL

Parasite Cleanse

Whole-body parasite & worm clearing

BY **DIANA M. DRAKE, BCTN** · DMD NATURAL MEDICINE

① LABS — OPTIONAL

DOCTOR'S DATA

3-Day Parasitology

Keep in mind that just because a parasite lab comes back negative does **not** mean that you don't have them. Everyone has parasites, and parasite cleansing is essential.

② SUPPLEMENTS

DR. DALE'S · LIQUID

Bio-Tox Total Parasite

DOSE 5 droppers full daily.

DR. DALE'S

Para-Pro Capsules

DOSE 2 capsules with each meal. 6 days on, 1 day off — three weeks on, 1 week off.

☽ Make sure you are **ON** the remedy during the full moon each round.

DR. DALE'S

Colon Pro

DOSE 1–3 capsules with meals. If diarrhea occurs, reduce the dose.

③ PROTOCOL NOTES — DURATION & MAINTENANCE

Follow this protocol for **6 months straight**, cycling **3 weeks on and 1 week off**. Always make sure you are **ON** the protocol during the full moon, as parasites are more active at that time. After the first 6 months, repeat for **30–120 days, or twice yearly,** as maintenance.

This protocol is provided for educational purposes and is intended for patients under the care of a qualified practitioner. It is not a substitute for individualized medical advice, diagnosis, or treatment. Do not begin, stop, or adjust any supplement without consulting your provider, particularly if you are pregnant, nursing, taking medications, or managing a medical condition.

CLINICAL PROTOCOL · 100% NATURAL

Whole Body Detox

Liver, kidney, lymph, colon & environmental toxin support

BY **DIANA M. DRAKE, BCTN** · DMD NATURAL MEDICINE

① LABS — OPTIONAL

MOSAIC DIAGNOSTICS

ToxDetect Profile

DOCTOR'S DATA

Hair Elements Test

Add **Dr. Dale's Bio-Tox Total Metals** only if heavy metals are present on the hair analysis.

② SUPPLEMENTS

DR. DALE'S

Liver Detox and Support

DOSE 3 caps 3×/day with meals. 5 days on, 2 days off.

DR. DALE'S

Whole Body Immune Pro

DOSE 3 caps 3×/day with meals. 5 days on, 2 days off.

DR. DALE'S

Kidney Pro

DOSE 3 caps 3×/day with meals. 5 days on, 2 days off.

DR. DALE'S

Colon Pro

DOSE 1–2 caps with each meal.

DR. DALE'S

Bio-Tox Total Metals

DOSE 5 droppers full daily.

DR. DALE'S

Lymph Detox Plus Drops

DOSE 5 drops in the AM & PM, Monday–Friday only. No caffeine.

DR. DALE'S

Bio-Tox Environmental Detox + Glyphosate

DOSE 5 droppers full per day.

③ PROTOCOL NOTES

DIET DURING THE DETOX

For best results during detoxing, do not consume animal products (flesh, dairy, or butter) or processed grains of any kind (corn, wheat, etc.). Only whole organic grains are okay — for example, quinoa in a salad or whole brown rice in a rice-and-veggie bowl. No pasta, bread, or gluten.

This protocol is provided for educational purposes and is intended for patients under the care of a qualified practitioner. It is not a substitute for individualized medical advice, diagnosis, or treatment. Do not begin, stop, or adjust any supplement without consulting your provider, particularly if you are pregnant, nursing, taking medications, or managing a medical condition.

CLINICAL PROTOCOL · 100% NATURAL

Candida Cleanse / Fungal Detox

Clearing candida, yeast & fungal overgrowth

BY **DIANA M. DRAKE, BCTN** · DMD NATURAL MEDICINE

① RECOMMENDED LABS

MOSAIC LABS · URINE

MycoTOX Panel

② SUPPLEMENTS

DR. DALE'S

Bio-Tox Total Fungal

DOSE 5 droppers full per day.

QUICKSILVER SCIENTIFIC

Ultra Binder Caps

DOSE 4 capsules once daily with water, 30 minutes before OR 2 hours after any meal.

A "binder" acts as an absorbent for what we call "die-off" — dead fungal/candida particles — and helps flush them from the body via the colon.

DR. DALE'S

Bio Film Detox

DOSE 1 capsule 20 minutes before each meal.

DR. DALE'S

Whole Body Immune Pro

DOSE 2 caps 3×/day with meals.

③ RECOMMENDED PEPTIDES

REJUVATIDE PEPTIDES

REJUVATIDE PEPTIDES · IMMUNE SUPPORT

Thymosin Alpha-1 — 10 mg

DOSE **ACUTE INFECTION (< 2 YEARS):** 10 units once daily, 5 days on, 2 days off. Sub-Q.
CHRONIC INFECTION (> 2 YEARS): 15 units AM or PM, twice weekly, 8 weeks on, 8 weeks off.
Reconstitute with 1 mL bacteriostatic water.

④ EVENING FOOT SOAK

15 DAYS

Hydrogen Peroxide Foot Soak

HOW In the evenings, soak your feet for 30 minutes before bed in warm water and hydrogen peroxide — 1 part peroxide to 3 parts water.

This helps rid the body of toxins, fungus, and bacteria.

⑤ ANTI-FUNGAL DIET

THESE ARE THE FOODS THAT FEED CANDIDA & FUNGAL INFECTION

✗ 100% ELIMINATE

- Sugar & sweeteners (honey, sweets, soda, maple syrup, etc.)
- Dairy (the lactose is a form of sugar)
- All fruit **except berries, lemons & limes**
- Fermented foods, including kombucha, kimchi, sauerkraut (these further ferment yeast)
- Vinegar: pickles, condiments, salad dressings

✓ FOCUS ON — YOU CAN EAT

PROTEIN
Meat, eggs, protein powder. Always organic.

COMPLEX CARBOHYDRATES
Non-starchy veggies — all greens, tomatoes, peppers, etc.

FRUIT
Frozen berries (freezing removes the mold), lemons, grapefruit. No other fruit.

BEANS
Black & pinto. Chili is a great meal.

GRAINS
Old-fashioned oatmeal is the ONLY grain you can have.

FATS
Olive oil, coconut, almonds, peanut butter (stir in a little colloidal silver to kill mold). If you want cheese, eat goat cheese.

⑥ PROTOCOL NOTES

After you have finished the detox, you may start repopulating with **Dr. Dale's Microbiome Terrain Pro** and an acidophilus probiotic.

This protocol is provided for educational purposes and is intended for patients under the care of a qualified practitioner. It is not a substitute for individualized medical advice, diagnosis, or treatment. Do not begin, stop, or adjust any supplement or peptide without consulting your provider, particularly if you are pregnant, nursing, taking medications, or managing a medical condition.

DR. DALE'S PROTOCOL · 100% NATURAL

72-Hour Gallbladder Flush

A 3-day liver & gallbladder cleanse

BY **DIANA M. DRAKE, BCTN** · DMD NATURAL MEDICINE

⚠ **Before you begin — two safety essentials.**

1. Do not flush a known stone larger than 5–6 mm (confirmed on an ultrasound).

2. Absolutely no caffeine — the gallbladder tinctures will not work in the body if caffeine is present. If you drink caffeine daily, wean off slowly the week before by going down 10% each day, or you may give yourself a headache and feel unwell.

Timing. Start the prep on **Friday & Saturday**; the flush itself is done **Saturday evening**, with the elimination on **Sunday**. If you do not eat 3 meals per day, only take the protocol during the 2 mealtimes that you eat.

① DAYS 1 & 2 — DETOX & STARVE THE GALLBLADDER

FRI & SAT

DR. DALE'S

Kidney Pro

DOSE 3 capsules 3×/day with meals.

DR. DALE'S

Liver Detox and Support

DOSE 3 capsules 3×/day with meals.

DR. DALE'S

Whole Body Immune Pro

DOSE 3 capsules 3×/day with meals.

DR. DALE'S

Colon Pro

DOSE 1–2 capsules with meals, to bowel tolerance. If diarrhea occurs, reduce the dose.

DR. DALE'S #2 GALLBLADDER

MBM or NER Homeopathic Remedy

DOSE 5 drops under the tongue between breakfast and dinner (on an empty stomach).

DIET FOR DAYS 1 & 2

Eat very light meals, 3 per day — all organic, healthy, **fiber-based** meals with fruits, veggies, beans, legumes, and whole grains. You **cannot consume any fat or oil** during this process.

Avoid: meat, dairy, butter, nuts, olive oil and any kind of oil (steam foods to cook instead), salad dressing, potato chips, etc.

Apple juice drink: Mix ½ oz of Dr. Dale's **Ortho Phos** into one quart of organic unfiltered apple juice diluted with purified water. Drink an entire quart each day, slowly throughout the day.

② SATURDAY EVENING — THE FLUSH

DAY OF THE FLUSH

During the day: eat a light breakfast and lunch. Continue the apple juice drink (½ oz Ortho Phos in a quart of diluted organic unfiltered apple juice).

Supplements today: take Kidney Pro, Liver Detox and Support, Colon Pro & Whole Body Immune Pro at the same doses, but timed — **upon rising, with lunch**, and **one hour before bedtime**. Take the #2 Gallbladder homeopathic (5 drops under the tongue) between breakfast and dinner, on an empty stomach.

6:00 PM	Take 1 teaspoon of Baja Gold Sea Salt dissolved in ¾ cup warm water. You may follow this with freshly squeezed grapefruit and lemon juice.
8:00 PM	Repeat the 6:00 PM steps (salts and juice).
8:30–9:30 PM (RIGHT BEFORE BED)	**Blend and drink** ½ cup warm, unrefined virgin olive oil with ¾ cup organic fresh-squeezed lemon, lime, or grapefruit juice. Do not heat the oil in the microwave — warm it gently on the stove (place the bottle in a pot of warm water to warm it safely).
IMMEDIATELY AFTER	**Go to bed and lie on your RIGHT side for 30 minutes.** You may then lie on your back or stay on your side. Do not get up — go to sleep.

③ DAY 3, SUNDAY — ELIMINATION

STOP ALL CAPSULES & DROPS

6:00 AM	Take 1 teaspoon of Baja Gold Sea Salt dissolved in ¾ cup warm water. You can go back to bed if you'd like.
8:00 AM	Repeat with the salt water.
10:00 AM	Eat a light breakfast of watermelon or berries (organic). Then a light lunch and a normal dinner.
THROUGHOUT THE DAY	**Stay close to the toilet** — your body will flush today via the colon, likely multiple times.

④ MAINTENANCE PROGRAM

2 WEEKS OFF, THEN 5 ON / 2 OFF

DR. DALE'S #2 GALLBLADDER

MBM Homeopathic

DOSE 5 drops 3×/day, 3 days per week, between meals.

Continues to detoxify the gallbladder and the emotion "resentment."

DR. DALE'S

Whole Body Immune Pro

DOSE 3 caps 2×/day, 5 days per week, on an empty stomach.

DR. DALE'S

Liver Detox and Support

DOSE 3 caps 2×/day, 5 days per week, on an empty stomach.

To cleanse and purify the liver.

DR. DALE'S

Kidney Pro

DOSE 3 caps 2×/day, 5 days per week, on an empty stomach.

To cleanse and purify the kidneys.

DR. DALE'S

Colon Pro

DOSE 1–2 caps, once or twice daily, at the same time as Whole Body Immune Pro, on an empty stomach.

To cleanse and purify the colon.

⑤ WHAT TO EXPECT

1. After the flush, you may experience gallstone detoxification for the next 3 days, with watery stools in the morning.

2. Some people report slight-to-moderate **nausea** from the olive oil & lemon juice cocktail; it slowly dissipates by the time you sleep. If the oil induces vomiting, do not repeat that step now — wait a week and repeat. This occurs very rarely.

3. Those who chronically suffer from gallstones, biliousness, backaches, or nausea occasionally find small **gallstone-type objects** in the stool the next day — green and brown, pea-sized, irregular, sometimes gelatinous, ranging from grape-seed to cherry-seed size. If there seem to be many, **repeat the flush in 90 days**. Bile ducts may also contain cholesterol crystals (which don't form stones) — shiny crystals floating on top of the water.

4. Expect one bowel movement per meal consumed. Initially (for 3–4 days), stools may occur more frequently — 4 or even 5 times per day — as the body throws off old waste.

⑥ FOODS TO ELIMINATE

DURING THE PROTOCOL

Vinegar · Dairy products · Fermented foods · Fried food · All oils · Desserts · Breads · Junk food · Sugar · Animal products · Alcohol · Caffeine

Water intake: aim for 1 gallon per day. Remember, when we cleanse, not only the junk comes out but so does the good — vitamins and minerals — so eat well, with lots of fruits and veggies, and cut out animal products, processed carbs, and sugar during the cleanse.

⑦ FRESH JUICE RECIPE

OPTIONAL · UP TO 16 OZ/DAY

Organic juice is an adjunct to this flush — highly recommended for best results, but not required. Drink up to **16 oz per day** (please do not exceed this). If you don't own a juicer, don't feel pressured to buy one just for this cleanse.

If you have diabetes or blood sugar problems, eliminate the apple and the carrot.

1 medium carrot · Kale · ½ tsp ginger root · 1 medium beet · Cucumber · ¼ apple · Dandelion · Parsley · 5 sprigs cilantro · Collard greens · Celery · Garlic

⑧ SHOPPING LIST

DR. DALE'S / PRACTICE

- Liver Detox and Support
- Kidney Pro
- Colon Pro
- Whole Body Immune Pro
- MBM or NER Gallbladder Homeopathic Tincture
- Ortho Phos

FROM THE NATURAL GROCERY STORE

- Baja Gold Sea Salt
- Organic unfiltered apple juice
- Organic extra virgin olive oil
- Fresh grapefruit to juice (or lemon / lime)

⑨ PROTOCOL NOTES

1. The gallbladder flush should be done **once yearly** as proper maintenance for the body.
2. If stones are known and/or common, repeat the flush **every 6 weeks** until they clear, then **twice yearly** as maintenance.
3. **Do not attempt to flush a known stone larger than 5–6 mm** (confirmed on an ultrasound).

This protocol is provided for educational purposes and is intended for patients under the care of a qualified practitioner. It is not a substitute for individualized medical advice, diagnosis, or treatment. Do not attempt a gallbladder flush if you have a known stone larger than 5–6 mm, a history of gallbladder attacks, bile-duct obstruction, or other biliary disease; seek medical care for severe abdominal pain, fever, or jaundice. Consult your provider before beginning, particularly if you are pregnant, nursing, diabetic, taking medications, or managing a medical condition.

CLINICAL PROTOCOL · 100% NATURAL

Water Fasting

What happens in the body, hour by hour — with prep & refeeding

BY **DIANA M. DRAKE, BCTN** · DMD NATURAL MEDICINE

① THE FASTING TIMELINE — BENEFITS BY HOURS FASTED

0–24 HRS Metabolic Reset

- **Blood sugar regulation:** insulin levels drop; the body begins switching from glucose to fat for energy.
- **Digestive rest:** the GI tract rests; inflammatory cytokines decrease.
- **Hormone response:** growth hormone increases slightly to preserve lean muscle.
- **Cellular hydration:** the body conserves water and electrolytes.

24–48 HRS Ketosis & Autophagy Activation

- **Ketosis begins:** the liver starts converting fat to ketones for brain and muscle fuel.
- **Autophagy initiated:** cells start clearing out damaged proteins, organelles, and toxins.
- **Mitochondrial cleanup:** early mitochondrial repair and turnover begin.
- **Mental clarity:** many report improved focus and reduced anxiety as ketones rise.
- **Inflammation reduction:** pro-inflammatory markers (e.g., IL-6, CRP) start decreasing.

48–72 HRS Deep Autophagy & Immune Reset

- **Stem cell activation:** bone marrow begins releasing new immune cells.
- **Intestinal healing:** mucosal inflammation reduces; gut permeability improves.
- **Insulin sensitivity:** resets significantly; metabolic pathways recalibrate.
- **Growth hormone surge:** GH may rise 300–500%, preserving muscle tissue.
- **Neuroprotection:** ketone bodies (especially β-hydroxybutyrate) protect neurons and enhance BDNF.

72–96+ HRS Regeneration Phase

- **Immune system renewal:** damaged immune cells are cleared and replaced with new, more efficient ones.
- **Systemic autophagy peak:** deep organ-level detox and cellular recycling.
- **Inflammation reset:** arthritis, allergy, and autoimmune markers can drop.
- **Stem cell proliferation:** triggered for repair in gut lining, skin, and brain tissue.
- **Emotional / mental clarity:** commonly reported, due to stabilized ketone energy and neurotransmitter balance.

② BEFORE YOU BEGIN — CLEAR THE COLON

Before you begin your fast you must clear your colon. This gets all of the stool out of your large intestine — otherwise you will have rotting stool sitting inside while you fast, because the colon stops moving.

1. **Colon hydrotherapy / colonic** at a professional clinic, the morning of day 1.
2. **Smooth Move Tea, then a salt flush:** 2 tablespoons of Baja Gold Sea Salt in 16 oz of warm water. Drink it quickly and stay by the toilet. Repeat the salt flush each morning until the water coming out of your colon runs clear. Do not add anything else to the salt flush.
3. **Salt flush only:** repeat daily until the water coming out of your colon runs clear.

③ WATER QUALITY & MINERALIZATION

Each day, be sure to drink water that is pure and well-mineralized. The options below are ranked, with the most ideal at the top.

- BEST — Distilled water, made fresh by you or bought in glass. Do not buy plastic.
- 2ND — Pre-filtered, then reverse-osmosis water at the tap — not in plastic.
- 3RD — Spring water in glass.
- 4TH — Berkey (or otherwise well-filtered) water in your home, drunk from glass.

Mineralize your water: add ⅛ teaspoon of Baja Gold Sea Salt per 30 oz of water. You can also add lemon.

④ BREAKING THE FAST — WHAT TO EAT

DAY 1 — Homemade organic soups, fresh-pressed juice, a vegan protein shake, or coconut yogurt — nothing solid and no processed foods. Eat light; your stomach will be small.

DAY 2 — Well-steamed veggies, rice, avocado, berries, protein shake, soup, coconut yogurt. Today you can incorporate larger amounts of food.

DAY 3 — Return to normal-size, portioned meals. Ideally, stay on whole foods and avoid animal products and sugar for as long as you can.

⑤ PROTOCOL NOTES

When you are calculating your hours of fasting, the fast starts **after your last meal**.

This protocol is provided for educational purposes and is intended for patients under the care of a qualified practitioner. It is not a substitute for individualized medical advice, diagnosis, or treatment. Extended water fasting is not appropriate for everyone — it should be avoided by those who are pregnant or nursing, underweight, or who have diabetes, an eating disorder, or other medical conditions, and by those on medications affected by fasting. Longer fasts are best undertaken with medical supervision. Break your fast gradually as described, and stop and seek care for fainting, chest pain, confusion, or other concerning symptoms. Consult your provider before beginning.

CLINICAL PROTOCOL · 100% NATURAL

Heavy Metal Detox

Heal the gut first, then clear the metals

BY **DIANA M. DRAKE, BCTN** · DMD NATURAL MEDICINE

① RECOMMENDED LABS

DOCTOR'S DATA

Hair Analysis

Hair testing gives a longer-term picture of metal accumulation and body burden.

DOCTOR'S DATA

Toxic Metals Urine Test

Urine testing captures what the body is actively excreting, and pairs well with the hair analysis for a fuller picture.

⚠ **Very high metals may require supervised chelation.**
If heavy metals are highly out of range, metal chelation may be necessary and should be performed under the supervision of a specialist or wellness professional with this specific experience. A protocol of this caliber will likely include a series of heavy-metal chelation IVs and physical detoxification such as infrared sauna.

② PHASE 1 — HEAL THE GUT FIRST

Before you remove metals from the system, it is important to heal the gut. Follow the path below that matches your situation. You may fit more than one.

IF YOU SUFFER FROM CONSTIPATION

- Increase fiber-based foods.
- Increase purified, mineralized water.
- **60 days of Dr. Dale's Microbiome Terrain Pro**, working up to 2 capsules with every meal and 2 capsules AM & PM on an empty stomach. Reduce if gas increases.
- **60 days of Dr. Dale's Digest Pro.**
- **Magnesium Oxide** to help the colon move.

IF YOU HAVE FOOD SENSITIVITIES OR TESTED POSITIVE FOR LEAKY GUT

- Remove all food sensitivities from your diet.
- **Dr. Dale's Digest Pro** in the AM, PM, and with every meal.
- **Dr. Dale's Microbiome Terrain Pro** in the AM, PM, and with every meal.
- **Dr. Dale's Systemic Enzyme Pro.**

> Extreme cases may require more support.

IF YOU SUFFER FROM PARASITES OR CANDIDA

- Follow the **Parasite Cleanse** and/or **Candida Cleanse** protocols in this book to balance those specific pathogens.

IF YOU SUFFER FROM GAS AND BLOATING

- Test for food sensitivities and remove them.
- Test for parasites and candida, and run those protocols if present.
- **60 days of Dr. Dale's Microbiome Terrain Pro.**
- **60 days of Dr. Dale's Digest Pro.**

③ PHASE 2 — THE METAL DETOX

Only once your gut is **no longer permeable and is functioning normally** can you run this metal detox.

DR. DALE'S
Bio-Tox Total Metals

> DOSE Follow the directions on the bottle.

DR. DALE'S
Full Body Detox

> DOSE Liver Detox and Support, Kidney Pro & Whole Body Immune Pro: 3 caps, 3 times daily with meals. Monday–Friday only.

DR. DALE'S
Colon Pro

> DOSE 1–2 capsules daily with meals, to your bowel tolerance. 7 days per week.

DR. DALE'S
Hepatic Glutathione Pathway

> DOSE 3 caps with breakfast.

Opens the liver pathway to detox metals.

QUICKSILVER SCIENTIFIC

Ultra Binder Capsules

DOSE Follow the directions on the bottle.

④ PROTOCOL NOTES

Glutathione and Vitamin C IVs are very beneficial as well. Run this protocol for **60–90 days, then re-test.**

This protocol is provided for educational purposes and is intended for patients under the care of a qualified practitioner. It is not a substitute for individualized medical advice, diagnosis, or treatment. Heavy-metal chelation, and any IV therapy, must be performed under qualified medical supervision. Heal the gut before beginning metal removal. Do not begin, stop, or adjust any supplement or therapy without consulting your provider, particularly if you are pregnant, nursing, taking medications, or managing a medical condition.

Chapter 6
Immunity

Where is your immune system located? Your immune system is a series of processes and channels that work together to rid your body of junk or "non-self". The more junk you acquire, the more the system gets backed up and starts to respond by alerting you with a series of warnings. Warnings are symptoms that something is not working. They can last for a short period of time; this is called acute. If the symptoms have gone on for longer than 2 years this is considered chronic. For example, a stuffy nose during a cold versus continuing to get sinus infections frequently. Each of us is our own bio individual. Meaning what one person reacts to - you may not. Think of a group of people standing in a field of grass in the spring. Some enjoy the sun and fresh air while others suffer allergy attacks. It is your individual terrain and current burden on your immune system that allows some to suffer and others to go unscathed.

The answer to allergies in Western Medicine is a suite of over the counter and prescription drugs called "antihistamines". Antihistamines stop the histamine response in your body that causes your negative reaction to ragweed, pollen and dust. This school of thought, however, does not ever help the body clear the allergen. It simply stops you from suffering by stopping the symptoms. When you take a drug for allergies, you are failing to help rid your immune system of the immense burden it is under - especially in the liver and lymphatic system. Detoxification is a major pillar of immune health from a naturopathic perspective. Keeping the liver and lymphatics clean can help lessen your reaction to histamine-causing particles.

Homeopathic remedies are also very valuable here. A type of homeopathic preparation for allergies is called an "isopathic" remedy. An isopathic remedy is made from the very substance that causes the reaction. It is delivered to the body in a more diluted and potentized version allowing the body to cancel out that frequency due to the theory of "like cures like". Snake venom is also used in the antidote; homeopathic allergy remedies deliver the same type of antidote for specific allergies. These remedies can be broad spectrum or contain specific ingredients.

Seasonal colds and flu can be completely avoided with proper detoxification and nutrition. You truly don't ever need to be sick. Your body expressing a cold or flu is simply a forced detox when it has become overburdened with toxins and is depleted of proper nutrition. Groups of people often get sick at the same time when they have been exposed to something environmentally. This includes a whole family getting sick at the same time. Families eat the same diet, drink the same water and breathe the same air from home. It is a common myth that your children "bring home" colds and flu's once they get back to school. Although I absolutely recognize that kids all get sick when they go back to school, let's look at what else is potentially going on here. Schools are often very old, poorly ventilated buildings cleaned with toxic chemical cleaners by the janitorial staff. They also have unfiltered tap water and serve terrible food. The school atmosphere puts your child under a ton of stress while they bathe in fluorescent lighting and EMF's all day long without rest. If your child is not properly hydrated, detoxed and lacks nutrition, their immune system is going to run down, and they are going to get sick. Period. This has absolutely nothing to do with catching it from other kids. The other kids are simply subject to the same environment as your child. Your child doesn't bring home germs - you and everyone around you already have a complex system of microbes, including viruses, bacteria, parasites and fungus. If you are getting sick at the same time as your children then I am suggesting you also are stressed, toxic, dehydrated and improperly nourished.

If this sounds like you and your household, I encourage you to put your family on my "Family Immune Plan" for an entire year and watch the decrease in the frequency of cold and flu incidents. Truly, you should not get sick more than once every few years if you are healthy, and I am speaking from experience. I used to get sick 5-8 times per year like clockwork when I went on a plane or when the seasons changed. After I started running these immune protocols - I simply do not get sick anymore except for if I have a known exposure to debris that gets into my sinuses or lungs. For example, if I am at a hotel and I can smell the HVAC system and see the unclean vents - I already know that I am in for it. But I know it's not from a germ - it's from my body becoming overburdened with particles of dust and God knows what in my respiratory system. When this happens, I spend the following 72 hours trying to clear those pathways. During this time, I am not lying up in bed - I simply have a runny nose and a cough. But it was not always that way for me. Historically, getting sick used to take me out for days at a time during which I could not work and could barely function. Looking back, I don't even remember what it felt like to be sick in that manner. "Never Be Sick Again" by Raymond Francis is a great read if you would like to learn more about this concept.

"Auto-Immune" disease is a western medical concept where you are taught that your body attacks itself for no known reason. In natural medicine, there is always a root cause at play. I know from testing hundreds of diseased thyroids that most people's thyroids are full of toxic bromine and chlorine rather than iodine which is the proper fuel for the thyroid. If a tissue is toxic, this is the perfect invitation for the immune system to go to work trying to remove said toxin. When it cannot - it gets stuck in overactive mode or what is called auto-immune disease. Many immune issues can be avoided if you simply stop taking vaccines and stop giving them to children and dogs. Immunity issues can then further be avoided by proper nutrition and detoxification. There are truly only two causes of disease. Too much of something your body doesn't need (toxemia) and/or not enough of something it does need (proper nutrition).

While I am focusing on regular immune protocols for this chapter, I highly encourage anyone with an auto-immune disorder to work with a naturopath that specializes in your specific condition or at least has experience in the auto-immune realm with a similar philosophy to what I have laid out here. This philosophy is referred to as terrain theory - versus germ theory which is the basis for the Western model that I speak about earlier in the book.

CLINICAL PROTOCOL · 100% NATURAL

Family Immune Protocol

Everyday immune support for adults & children

BY **DIANA M. DRAKE, BCTN** · DMD NATURAL MEDICINE

Detox quarterly — refer to the detox protocols in the detox section. For kids, lower the dose based on their weight; the standard dosages given are for a 150-pound person, so adjust accordingly.

① STOP EATING SUGAR AT HOME

Sugar can be an occasional treat if you are out, but it should be **100% eliminated in the home**. This includes:

- ✗ **Soda** — *use Zevia, Spindrift, or Culture Pop instead*
- ✗ **Store-bought juices** — *use pure Thailand coconut water instead (check for added sugar)*
- ✗ **Corn syrup** of any kind
- ✗ **Yogurt** with added sugar
- ✗ **Granola and cereals**
- ✗ **Bars and packaged snacks**
- ✗ **Halloween candy**

② SUPPLEMENTS — ADULTS

PURE ENCAPSULATIONS · 1,000 MG ASCORBIC ACID CAPS

Vitamin C

DOSE 3,000 mg per meal, three times per day.

Zinc

DOSE 30 mg per day.

Vitamin D

DOSE 5,000 IU per day (may increase to 10,000 IU in winter if in a cold climate).

Please make sure to take **vitamin K** while taking vitamin D.

Magnesium Glycinate

DOSE 500 mg per day.

PROIMMUNE

ProImmune Powder

DOSE 1 scoop daily, dissolved directly in the mouth.

③ SUPPLEMENTS — CHILDREN

MY KIND ORGANICS

Whole Food Vitamin C

DOSE 8 sprays per day; 12 sprays per day during the winter months.

PROIMMUNE

ProImmune Powder

DOSE ¼–⅓ scoop daily, dissolved in the mouth, depending on the child's weight.

AGE	ZINC (PICOLINATE PREFERRED)	VITAMIN D (DROPS OR CHEWABLE)	MAGNESIUM GLYCINATE
1–3	2–3 mg/day	600 IU/day	80 mg/day
4–8	5 mg/day	600–1,000 IU/day	120–160 mg/day
9–13	8 mg/day	1,000 IU/day	150–200 mg/day
14–18	Girls 9 mg · Boys 11 mg/day	1,000 IU/day	300–400 mg/day

This protocol is provided for educational purposes and is intended for patients under the care of a qualified practitioner. It is not a substitute for individualized medical advice, diagnosis, or treatment. Children's doses are general guidelines and should be adjusted for weight and confirmed with your pediatric provider. Do not begin, stop, or adjust any supplement without consulting your provider, particularly if a family member is pregnant, nursing, taking medications, or managing a medical condition.

CLINICAL PROTOCOL · 100% NATURAL

Chronic Sinus Infections

Immune, antimicrobial & sinus support

BY **DIANA M. DRAKE, BCTN** · DMD NATURAL MEDICINE

Detox every quarter using the Dr. Dale Whole Body Detox Kit (also see the detoxification protocols).

① RECOMMENDED PEPTIDE — REJUVATIDE PEPTIDES

REJUVATIDE PEPTIDES · IMMUNE SUPPORT

Thymosin Alpha-1 — 10 mg

> DOSE Reconstitute with 1 mL bacteriostatic water. Chronic infection: 15 units in the AM or PM, twice weekly. 8 weeks on, 8 weeks off. Sub-Q injection.

Once the infection clears, you can stay on this dose as maintenance. If an active infection comes back, switch to the active-infection dose.

② NASAL & SINUS CARE

Nasal Colloidal Silver Spray

> DOSE 2 sprays in each nostril several times daily.

Can be used on an active infection to help reduce microbes. At the onset of a sore throat, spray into the throat as well as the nose.

FLAVENT RELIEF

Nasal Relief Sinus Spray

> DOSE Use as directed to relieve congestion and support the nasal passages.

Neti Pot — traditional ceramic

Use to keep the sinus passages clear and moisturized.

③ SUPPLEMENTS

DR. DALE'S

Allercyl Airborne

DOSE 5 drops 2×/day. 5 days on, 2 days off. No caffeine.

PROIMMUNE

ProImmune Powder

DOSE 1 scoop daily, dissolved directly in the mouth.

This protocol is provided for educational purposes and is intended for patients under the care of a qualified practitioner. It is not a substitute for individualized medical advice, diagnosis, or treatment. Use only sterile, distilled, or previously boiled water in a neti pot. Seek medical care for high fever, severe facial pain or swelling, or symptoms that worsen or do not improve. Do not begin, stop, or adjust any peptide or supplement without consulting your provider, particularly if you are pregnant, nursing, taking medications, or managing a medical condition.

CLINICAL PROTOCOL · 100% NATURAL

Chronic Viral Overburden

A cumulative 3-phase immune, antiviral & cellular-repair protocol

BY **DIANA M. DRAKE, BCTN** · DMD NATURAL MEDICINE

PHASE 1		PHASE 2		PHASE 3
Immune Regulation Weeks 1–4	+	**Anti-Viral** Weeks 3–10	+	**Mitochondrial & Cellular Repair** Weeks 4–16

Phases are cumulative. When a new phase starts, continue taking all the items from the previous phase.

① PHASE 1 — IMMUNE REGULATION — WEEKS 1–4

REJUVATIDE PEPTIDES · IMMUNE SUPPORT

Thymosin Alpha-1

DOSE Reconstitute with 1 mL bacteriostatic water. Chronic infection: 15 units in the AM or PM, twice weekly. 8 weeks on, 8 weeks off. Sub-Q injection.

Vitamin D

DOSE 5,000 units daily.

Vitamin K should be taken alongside D for proper absorption.

Zinc Picolinate

DOSE 15–30 mg daily.

DR. DALE'S

Nano-Ionic Selenium

DOSE 30 drops daily.

PROIMMUNE

ProImmune Powder

DOSE 1 scoop daily, dissolved directly in the mouth.

② PHASE 2 — ANTI-VIRAL — INTRODUCE DURING WEEKS 3–10

+ **Continue everything from Phase 1.**

Monolaurin ECOLOGICAL FORMULAS / CARDIOVASCULAR RESEARCH	600 mg, 2–3×/day
Olive Leaf Extract PURE ENCAPSULATIONS	500 mg, 2×/day
Cat's Claw PURE ENCAPSULATIONS	500 mg, 2×/day
L-Lysine (amino acid) PURE ENCAPSULATIONS	1,000 mg, 1–2×/day

③ PHASE 3 — MITOCHONDRIAL & CELLULAR REPAIR — WEEKS 4–16

+ **Continue everything from Phases 1 & 2.**

CoQ10 (ubiquinol) PURE ENCAPSULATIONS	100–200 mg daily
Acetyl-L-Carnitine PURE ENCAPSULATIONS	500–1,000 mg daily
Alpha-Lipoic Acid PURE ENCAPSULATIONS	300–600 mg daily
B-Complex (methylated) BIOTICS RESEARCH	Daily

INJECTABLE COENZYME

NAD+ — 500 mg

> DOSE Reconstitute the bottle to the top with bacteriostatic water. Inject 200 units into sub-Q fat once daily for 5 days, then reduce to 100 units twice weekly.

INJECTABLE ANTIOXIDANT

Glutathione — 1,500 mg bottle

> DOSE Reconstitute with 3 mL bacteriostatic water. Inject 300 units into sub-Q fat during midday, 3 days per week. 8 weeks on, 4 weeks off.

④ DIETARY RECOMMENDATIONS

✗ Sugar ✗ Caffeine ✗ Alcohol ✗ Gluten ✗ Dairy

Be sure to get plenty of **protein**, and be sure to **mineralize** your water.

This protocol is provided for educational purposes and is intended for patients under the care of a qualified practitioner. It is not a substitute for individualized medical advice, diagnosis, or treatment. Injectable peptides, NAD+, and glutathione should be used only under qualified medical supervision. Do not begin, stop, or adjust any peptide, injectable, or supplement without consulting your provider, particularly if you are pregnant, nursing, taking medications, or managing a medical condition.

ACUTE PROTOCOL · 10 DAYS · 100% NATURAL

Emergency Cold & Flu

A short, intensive 10-day immune protocol

BY **DIANA M. DRAKE, BCTN** · DMD NATURAL MEDICINE

① SUPPLEMENTS — 10 DAYS

Vitamin C PURE ENCAPSULATIONS	**5,000 mg, 3×/day**
Vitamin D THORNE	**80,000 IU/day**
Magnesium INTEGRATIVE THERAPEUTICS TRI-MAGNESIUM	**500 mg/day**
Zinc Picolinate DOUGLAS LABS Do not take on an empty stomach	**50 mg/day**

DR. DALE'S NAC PRO

N-Acetyl Cysteine (IF LUNG MUCUS IS PRESENT)

DOSE Add 3,000 mg per day.

DR. DALE'S

Cold Guard Plus Homeopathic Drops

DOSE 5 drops 3×/day.

② RECOMMENDED PEPTIDE — REJUVATIDE PEPTIDES

REJUVATIDE PEPTIDES · IMMUNE SUPPORT

Thymosin Alpha-1 — 10 mg

DOSE Reconstitute with 1 mL bacteriostatic water. Inject 20 units once daily for 5 days straight, then rest 2 days. Continue with 5 units, 5 days on / 2 days off, until you feel well again. Inject into sub-Q fat.

③ DIET

✗ **100% AVOID**

All dairy products | All sugar

WHAT TO EAT

Stick to a diet of broths, soups, fruit, and lightly steamed veggies. If you are not hungry and feeling flu-like, at the very least be sure to drink **bone broth** and drink water with minerals added back.

④ THERAPIES

Iodine Bath

HOW Add ¼ cup of iodine to your bath and soak.

Hydrogen Peroxide Foot Bath

HOW Soak your feet for 30 minutes before bed, every night, in a solution of ¾ parts water to ¼ part hydrogen peroxide.

This protocol is provided for educational purposes and is intended for patients under the care of a qualified practitioner. It is not a substitute for individualized medical advice, diagnosis, or treatment. The high-dose vitamins here are intended only for short-term (10-day) acute use and should be supervised by your provider; high-dose vitamin D requires vitamin K and monitoring. Seek medical care for difficulty breathing, chest pain, high or persistent fever, or symptoms that worsen. Do not begin, stop, or adjust any peptide or supplement without consulting your provider, particularly if you are pregnant, nursing, taking medications, or managing a medical condition.

CLINICAL PROTOCOL · 100% NATURAL

Seasonal Allergies

Histamine, lymphatic & immune support

BY **DIANA M. DRAKE, BCTN** · DMD NATURAL MEDICINE

① SUPPLEMENTS & REMEDIES

DR. DALE'S · HOMEOPATHIC

Allercyl Airborne & Allercyl Breathe

DOSE 5 drops 2×/day, AM & PM. Monday–Friday only.

DR. DALE'S

Lymphatic Detox Plus

DOSE 5 drops 2×/day, AM & PM. Monday–Friday only.

DR. DALE'S

Whole Body Detox Kit

DOSE Liver Detox and Support, Kidney Pro & Whole Body Immune Pro: 3 caps, 3×/day with meals. 5 days on, 2 days off.

Run the detox for 90 days.

DR. DALE'S

Multi-Minerals with Silica

DOSE 30 drops per day.

PURE ENCAPSULATIONS · ASCORBIC ACID CAPS

Vitamin C

DOSE 3 caps, 3×/day with meals. If diarrhea occurs, reduce the dose.

DESIGNS FOR HEALTH

Quercetin & Nettles

DOSE 1 capsule 3×/day with meals.

② RECOMMENDED PEPTIDE

REJUVATIDE PEPTIDES

REJUVATIDE PEPTIDES · IMMUNE SUPPORT

Thymosin Alpha-1 — 10 mg

> DOSE Reconstitute with 2 mL bacteriostatic water. Inject into fatty tissue (stomach, back of arm, top of buttocks, or thigh), AM or PM.
>
> **IMMUNE SUPPORT:** 5 units, 1×/day, 5 days on, 2 days off.
>
> **CHRONIC INFECTION:** 15 units, 2 doses per week, 8 weeks on, 8 weeks off.

This is a **slower-working** remedy that builds over time and is **not** for immediate relief. It is for severe, chronic allergy issues rooted in more than just a histamine response.

> Begin with the **chronic** dose, then step down to **immune support**.

This protocol is provided for educational purposes and is intended for patients under the care of a qualified practitioner. It is not a substitute for individualized medical advice, diagnosis, or treatment. Seek immediate care for any signs of a severe allergic reaction, such as difficulty breathing or throat swelling. Do not begin, stop, or adjust any peptide or supplement without consulting your provider, particularly if you are pregnant, nursing, taking medications, or managing a medical condition.

Chapter 7
Pain

Chronic pain can significantly affect quality of life. Whether it results from injury, repetitive strain, degenerative changes, or an unclear underlying cause, persistent pain is often driven by ongoing inflammation and impaired tissue repair. When tissue remains in a prolonged inflammatory state, your body's natural healing processes can become dysregulated or incomplete.

Peptide therapy offers a targeted, biologically intelligent approach to support healing. Peptides are short chains of amino acids that act as cell-signaling molecules, instructing the body to activate its own repair, regeneration, and anti-inflammatory pathways rather than simply masking symptoms.

Two peptides that have been extensively studied for pain and tissue recovery are;

BPC-157 and TB-500:

- **BPC-157 (Body Protection Compound-157)** is a peptide derived from a naturally occurring protein in the gastric system. It has been shown to support **tendon, ligament, muscle, nerve, and gut healing,** while also modulating inflammation and improving blood flow to injured tissue. BPC-157 is commonly used in chronic pain states related to soft-tissue injury, joint pain, and post-surgical recovery.

- **TB-500 (Thymosin Beta-4 fragment)** plays a role in **cell migration, tissue regeneration, and inflammation control.** It supports actin regulation within cells, which is critical for tissue repair and remodeling. TB-500 is often used for broader, systemic healing, particularly when pain is associated with widespread inflammation, repetitive injury, or delayed recovery.

Both peptides have a growing body of preclinical and clinical research, with published studies available in peer-reviewed scientific literature. When used appropriately, they may help shift the body out of chronic inflammation and back into a state of active repair, offering a regenerative option for individuals struggling with persistent pain.

CLINICAL PROTOCOL · 100% NATURAL

Bone Healing

Repair peptides, bone-building nutrients & topical support

BY **DIANA M. DRAKE, BCTN** · DMD NATURAL MEDICINE

① RECOMMENDED PEPTIDES

REJUVATIDE PEPTIDES · INJECT NEAR THE INJURY

REJUVATIDE PEPTIDES

BPC-157 — 10 mg

DOSE Add 2 mL bacteriostatic water. Inject 10 units twice daily near the injury, AM & PM, for 6 weeks — then take 2 weeks off.

REJUVATIDE PEPTIDES

TB-500 — 10 mg

DOSE Add 2 mL bacteriostatic water. Inject 100 units twice weekly in the AM near the injury, for 6 weeks — then take 3 weeks off.

REJUVATIDE PEPTIDES

GHK-Cu — 50 mg

DOSE Add 4 mL bacteriostatic water. Inject 8 units near the injury. 4 weeks on, 2 weeks off.

② SUPPLEMENTS

EIDON MINERALS

Bone Strong Formula

DOSE Take with water daily.

DR. DALE'S

Bio Age Erase — Collagen & Vitamin C powder

DOSE Daily, as directed.

DR. DALE'S

Vitamin D & K

DOSE 2 capsules daily.

PURE ENCAPSULATIONS

Additional Vitamin D (SHORT TERM · 20 DAYS)

DOSE An additional 10,000 IU of vitamin D per day, short term (20 days).

③ TOPICAL COMFREY POULTICE

ONCE THE SKIN IS INTACT

⚠ USE ONLY ONCE THE SKIN IS INTACT

HOW TO PREPARE

1. Use dried comfrey leaf or root.
2. Rehydrate it with warm water.
3. Apply as a thick paste over the area.
4. Cover with cloth; leave on 20–60 minutes.
5. Use 1–2× daily.

OR USE A TOPICAL COMFREY OINTMENT

- Christopher's Original Comfrey Ointment
- Nature's Own Herbals Comfrey Salve

④ DAILY GREEN SMOOTHIE

ALKALIZE & MINERALIZE

Drink a green smoothie daily to alkalize and mineralize the body. Blend:

Kale | Spinach | Blueberries | Cucumber | Key limes | Mint | Sea moss gel

This protocol is provided for educational purposes and is intended for patients under the care of a qualified practitioner. It is not a substitute for individualized medical advice, diagnosis, or treatment. Comfrey is for external use on intact skin only — do not apply to broken skin or open wounds, and do not take internally. High-dose vitamin D is intended for short-term use only, with vitamin K and monitoring. Fractures require appropriate medical evaluation and stabilization. Do not begin, stop, or adjust any peptide or supplement without consulting your provider, particularly if you are pregnant, nursing, taking medications, or managing a medical condition.

CLINICAL PROTOCOL · 100% NATURAL

Chronic Pain — Targeted

Injuries, post-surgery, chronic musculoskeletal / soft tissue, knees / hips / joints, spinal & disk issues

BY **DIANA M. DRAKE, BCTN** · DMD NATURAL MEDICINE

① RECOMMENDED PEPTIDES

REJUVATIDE · INJECT INTO OR NEAR THE PAIN

REJUVATIDE PEPTIDES

BPC-157 — 10 mg

DOSE Reconstitute with 2 mL bacteriostatic water. Inject 10–25 units once daily, 5 days on / 2 days off — 8 weeks on, 2 weeks off. Inject directly into or close to the area of pain.

REJUVATIDE PEPTIDES

TB-500 — 10 mg

DOSE Reconstitute with 2 mL bacteriostatic water. Inject 100 units twice weekly — 8 weeks on, 2 weeks off. Inject directly into or close to the area of pain.

② SUPPORTIVE CARE

MATCH TO YOUR INJURY TYPE

SOFT TISSUE If the injury is in the soft tissue, be sure you are taking a **collagen supplement** and **amino acids**.

JOINTS Support any joint issues with **MSM / Glucosamine** and **Hyaluronic Acid** capsules from Pure Encapsulations.

INJURY If it is an injury, also consider alternating **ice and heat** to keep blood flow to the area.

This protocol is provided for educational purposes and is intended for patients under the care of a qualified practitioner. It is not a substitute for individualized medical advice, diagnosis, or treatment. Peptide injections should be performed with proper technique and professional guidance, and targeted injections near a joint, the spine, or a surgical site warrant particular caution. Seek medical evaluation for new, severe, or worsening pain, numbness, weakness, or loss of function. Do not begin, stop, or adjust any peptide or supplement without consulting your provider, particularly if you are pregnant, nursing, taking medications, or managing a medical condition.

CLINICAL PROTOCOL · 100% NATURAL

Systemic Pain / Inflammation

For pain that is not specific to one area or injury — overall joint pain or whole-body inflammation

BY **DIANA M. DRAKE, BCTN** · DMD NATURAL MEDICINE

① RECOMMENDED PEPTIDES

REJUVATIDE · SUB-Q FAT

REJUVATIDE PEPTIDES

BPC-157 — 10 mg

DOSE Reconstitute with 2 mL bacteriostatic water. Inject 10–25 units once daily, 5 days on / 2 days off — 8 weeks on, 2 weeks off. Inject into the subcutaneous fat of the stomach, arm, or buttocks.

REJUVATIDE PEPTIDES

TB-500 — 10 mg

DOSE Reconstitute with 2 mL bacteriostatic water. Inject 100 units twice weekly — 8 weeks on, 2 weeks off. Inject into the subcutaneous fat of the stomach, arm, or buttocks.

② SUPPORTIVE CARE

JOINTS For inflamed joints, also support with **MSM / Glucosamine** and **Hyaluronic Acid** supplements from Pure Encapsulations.

DIET Eat an **anti-inflammatory diet** and remove your food sensitivities. **Sugar and gluten** especially should be cut out.

③ HERBS FOR JOINT PAIN

Other great herbs to help with joint pain:

Turmeric · Boswellia · Ginger · Willow Bark

This protocol is provided for educational purposes and is intended for patients under the care of a qualified practitioner. It is not a substitute for individualized medical advice, diagnosis, or treatment. Widespread or systemic pain and inflammation can have underlying causes that warrant medical evaluation. Some anti-inflammatory herbs (for example, willow bark) can interact with blood thinners and other medications. Do not begin, stop, or adjust any peptide, herb, or supplement without consulting your provider, particularly if you are pregnant, nursing, taking medications, or managing a medical condition.

Chapter 8
Skin & Hair Health

Hair Loss & Health - Women and men across the U.S. have been working with me on hair loss since I began my practice. Women tend to shed hair when they have a thyroid issue, high stress and go into menopause. Hair loss in men on the other hand has been linked to genetic predisposition and more recently to the over-abundance of a type of testosterone called DHT. It is important with hair loss cases to look at all the potential root casualties. The good news is, regardless of the reason, peptide-based hair loss protocols can be incredibly successful and are very easy to implement. Even if your hair is not thinning, this hair loss protocol will also support keeping the hair you have healthy and act as a preventative measure. It is important to note that the peptide needs to be used both topically and injected systemically into sub-cutaneous fat for best results.

Skin - At some point, every American suffers some sort of skin issue. From acne to unknown rashes and eczema, my extensive skin protocols are designed to heal skin issues by balancing the internal root causes - rather than focusing on topical treatments like a traditional dermatologist. In fact, dermatologists miss the mark completely when it comes to understanding skin problems. The skin is our biggest organ and is known in Chinese medicine as the third kidney. Each issue reflects a specific combination of internal imbalances taking place and they all have toxicity in common. This is why you will see detoxification in almost every skin protocol. I am also very diligent with targeted labs for each skin issue as this is a step often missed entirely when you go to the dermatologist.

As we discussed in the hormone chapter, PCOS and excess androgens that cause menstrual cycle and fertility issues in women are the same root causes that trigger hormonal acne in teenagers - boys too. These excess androgens (which are the wrong type of testosterone) get too high due to unhealthy diets high in sugars and carbohydrates (*in most cases). This is why I suggest taking a full hormone saliva test that also looks at adrenal health along with food sensitivities and a gut permeability test. In some cases, I also do a full microbiome stool panel if the case doesn't clear to 50% by the first 90 days.

Teens that grab antibiotics and Accutane for this condition are only causing further harm to your gut microbiome and health by avoiding the root cause and using drugs. I have seen very few cases who clear acne forever using only one round of an antibiotic or Accutane. This is typically a several-round treatment plan and eventually it tends to come back. I have also seen over time that Accutane can thin the skin and make it start to look translucent, making it very sensitive, easy to tear and reflects ageing poorly. Teen acne needs a combination of detoxification, hormone balancing and gut repair.

Eczema and Psoriasis are actually very similar to each other - the difference being that psoriasis has an auto-immune element to it and can have specific patterns on the body. But I can tell you they both have *extreme toxicity, immune imbalance* and *gut permeability* in common. When your body is not properly eliminating through the right channels, the next best exit is the skin. Eczema and Psoriasis are most simply described as an overburdened immune system expressing via the skin. Using topical steroids only stops your skin from expressing the toxins and keeps driving them back down into the body. This is actually very dangerous and can result in something called Topical Steroid

Withdrawal (TSW). In TSW your skin enters a continual inflammatory shedding cycle that can only be relieved by time. Additionally, your skin condition can come back with a vengeance - even worse than before, while your entire body turns into a crust that peels off - again. I have had many clients tell me they were nearly suicidal going through TSW.

Here's something you will never hear from a dermatologist, understanding if your skin condition is driven by TH-1 or TH-2 Immune response. The Th1 vs Th2 immune response reflects two different arms of adaptive immunity: Th1 is more inflammatory and cell-mediated (driven by cytokines like IFN-and TNF-), while Th2 is associated with humoral immunity, allergies, and IgE activity (driven by IL-4, IL-5, IL-13). In skin conditions, this balance is clinically relevant psoriasis is primarily dominant Th1/Th17, leading to rapid skin cell turnover and inflammatory plaque, whereas eczema (atopic dermatitis) is predominantly Th2 dominant, characterized by barrier dysfunction, elevated IgE, and allergic reactivity. Many patients, however, can exhibit immune dysregulation rather than pure dominance, with shifts between pathways depending on triggers, making immune-modulating strategies (rather than purely suppressive ones) more effective long term. For the protocols I am providing, we will assume TH-1 dominance with Psoriasis and TH-2 Dominance with eczema. Eczema is generally understood as an inflamed skin condition whereas Psoriasis has an extra immune element to it. Therefore, I refer to my protocols such as Dermal-Inflammation and Dermal-Inflammation with Immune Issues.

All skin conditions are best dealt with holistically, as natural protocols work with the body to assist with what your body needs to do to balance. When you suppress the excretion of toxins through your skin, I guarantee they will come out in other ways - turning into gut or asthma/lung issues. This is the stark difference between western and natural medicine. I began my career as an esthetician before I became a naturopath and have been working the longest on skin issues. They can affect so much from our self-esteem and confidence to how our body feels - especially when something is red and itching all over. Again, detoxification and proper gut permeability are important here as well as understanding food sensitivities and immune system balance. Each protocol will include recommended labs for best success. Labs on skin conditions are very important and not optional if you want to heal. It is very important that if a lab or multiple labs are recommended, that all of them are executed to understand the full picture.

CLINICAL PROTOCOL · 100% NATURAL

Hormonal Breakouts — Teens

Clearing teen acne from the inside out

BY **DIANA M. DRAKE, BCTN** · DMD NATURAL MEDICINE

Order of operations: begin with the 6-week natural anti-bacterial clean-up (Phase 1) **before** you start the foundational protocol (Phase 2).

① RECOMMENDED LABS

ACCESS MEDICAL LABS

OpenDx Supreme Saliva Hormone Test

Check for excess **androstenedione** and adrenal cortisol patterns.

PICK ONE TO FIT YOUR BUDGET

Food Sensitivity Testing

US BIOTEK

GI-Basic Profile

A map of the microbiome — this shows what needs to be corrected in the gut.

② PHASE 1 — ANTI-BACTERIAL CLEAN-UP

6 WEEKS · DO THIS FIRST

DR. DALE'S

Bio-Tox Total Bacteria Formula

DOSE 5 droppers full per day, AM or PM, on an empty stomach.

ANY BRAND

Oregon Grape Capsules

DOSE 500 mg with each meal.

SKIN NATUROPATHIC

Derma-Detox

DOSE 2–5 caps 3×/day with meals. If diarrhea occurs, reduce the dose.

Cleans out the skin, lymphatics, liver, colon, and kidneys. Take until the skin is 90% clear.

③ PHASE 2 — FOUNDATIONAL PROTOCOL

SKIN NATUROPATHIC

Hormonal Breakouts

> DOSE 2–4 capsules with each meal daily.

Balances androgens and blood sugar. Take until the skin is clear, then move to a maintenance dose of 1–2 caps with meals (or more if needed).

SKIN NATUROPATHIC

Biome Skin

> DOSE 1–2 caps with 1–3 meals per day.

Works on the gut lining and a healthy microbiome with spore-forming probiotics.

> If **leaky gut** is confirmed, use a higher dose — potentially up to 2 caps in the AM & PM on an empty stomach, plus with meals — then re-test for permeability in 90 days. Oral **BPC-157** peptides are also a good option to heal the gut.

> **Food sensitivities:** remove all food sensitivities that were flagged on the sensitivity test for 90 days, then re-test. As the gut heals, food sensitivities will lessen.

④ ADD-ON — IF ADRENAL CORTISOL WAS FLAGGED

IF ADRENAL CORTISOL PATTERNS WERE FLAGGED

- **Dr. Dale's Optimal Multi-Pro:** 2 caps with the first meal of the day.
- **Dr. Dale's Adaptogen Pro:** 2 caps in the AM and with the first meal of the day.

This protocol is provided for educational purposes and is intended for patients under the care of a qualified practitioner. It is not a substitute for individualized medical advice, diagnosis, or treatment. For teens, dosing and testing should be confirmed with a pediatric or qualified provider. Do not begin, stop, or adjust any supplement or peptide without consulting your provider, particularly if a medication or medical condition is involved.

CLINICAL PROTOCOL · 100% NATURAL

Peri-Oral Inflamed Rash

Inflamed rash around the nose & mouth

BY **DIANA M. DRAKE, BCTN** · DMD NATURAL MEDICINE

> This is generally caused by a **fungal infection in the small intestine** that must be cleared with a combination of both supplements and a strict diet. Removing food sensitivities during this time is important — although they are not the cause, they can be a trigger.

① RECOMMENDED LABS

ALLETESS MEDICAL LABS

Food Sensitivity Test

US BIOTEK

GI Basic Gut Panel

Checks for candida / fungal overgrowth in the gut — a common driver of peri-oral rash.

② PHASE 1 — REMOVE

RUN UNTIL THE SKIN IS 90% CLEAR

SKIN NATUROPATHIC

Rose Guard

> DOSE 2 in the AM & PM on an empty stomach.

SKIN NATUROPATHIC

Derma-Detox

> DOSE 3–4 capsules with meals until the skin clears. Reduce the dose if diarrhea occurs.

SKIN NATUROPATHIC

XMA Hista Clear (FOR ITCHING, IF PRESENT)

> DOSE 2–4 capsules with meals until you feel relief.

SKIN NATUROPATHIC

XMA Heat Clear (FOR IRRITATION & REDNESS)

> DOSE 2–4 capsules with meals until you feel relief.

DR. DALE'S

Bio-Film Detox

DOSE 1 capsule before each meal.

③ PHASE 2 — REPOPULATE & REBUILD

SKIN NATUROPATHIC

Biome Skin

DOSE 1 capsule with every meal.

KLAIRE LABS

Acidophilus Probiotic

DOSE Per manufacturer directions.

DR. DALE'S

Digest Pro

DOSE 2 in the AM & PM and 2 before each meal for the first 30 days of Phase 2, then reduce to 2 capsules before each meal.

④ DIET

✗ 100% ELIMINATE

Coffee · Sugar · Alcohol · Dairy · Spicy foods · Hot liquids · Gluten & processed grains

FOCUS ON

Whole, organic foods — lots of protein and veggies. Fruits should be limited to **berries only**, plus lemon in water.

⑤ TOPICAL RECOMMENDATIONS

Avoid stripping the skin with harsh, drying cleansers and soaps. Do not use anything with acids or a gritty scrub. **Oil or cream cleansers** will be much better for the face during this time. Use **coconut oil** as your moisturizer / treatment after cleansing.

This protocol is provided for educational purposes and is intended for patients under the care of a qualified practitioner. It is not a substitute for individualized medical advice, diagnosis, or treatment. A persistent or spreading facial rash should be evaluated to confirm the cause. Do not begin, stop, or adjust any supplement without consulting your provider, particularly if you are pregnant, nursing, taking medications, or managing a medical condition.

CLINICAL PROTOCOL · 100% NATURAL

PSO — Chronic Dermal Inflammation

Chronic skin inflammation with immune imbalance

BY **DIANA M. DRAKE, BCTN** · DMD NATURAL MEDICINE

> This common skin condition is the result of an **overburdened immune system** that expresses toxins via the skin, causing a reaction at the site. Removing food sensitivities during this time is important — although they are usually not the cause, they can be a trigger.

① RECOMMENDED LABS

ATTELESS LABS

Food Sensitivity Test

Available at www.SkinNaturopathics.com.

② PHASE 1 — DETOX

RUN UNTIL THE SKIN IS 90% CLEAR

SKIN NATUROPATHICS

Derma-Detox

> DOSE 3–4 capsules with meals until the skin clears. Reduce the dose if diarrhea occurs.

SKIN NATUROPATHICS

Rose Guard

> DOSE 2 in the AM & PM on an empty stomach. Run this for 2 rounds (2 bottles' worth).

To clear a fungal infection, which is likely present.

DR. DALE'S

Kidney Pro

> DOSE 2 caps with every meal.

SKIN NATUROPATHICS

XMA Hista Clear (FOR ITCHING, IF PRESENT)

> DOSE 2–4 capsules with meals until the skin clears to 90%.

SKIN NATUROPATHICS

XMA Heat Clear (FOR IRRITATION & REDNESS)

DOSE 2–4 capsules with meals until the skin clears to 90%.

③ PHASE 2 — IMMUNE & GUT BALANCE

SKIN NATUROPATHICS

Biome Skin

DOSE 1–2 capsules with every meal.

PURE ENCAPSULATIONS

TH-1 Supplement

DOSE 2 caps once or twice daily. Start with 2 and see how you feel.

Base the TH-1 vs TH-2 choice on your CytoDx immune-panel results, and bring it in **separately** so you can see how you feel.

PROIMMUNE

ProImmune Powder

DOSE 1 scoop daily, dissolved on the tongue.

DR. DALE'S

Digest Pro

DOSE 2 capsules in the AM & PM, and before every meal.

⏱ **After 6 weeks** on the above, you can bring in the peptides.

REJUVATIDE PEPTIDES · IMMUNE MODULATOR

Thymosin Alpha-1 — 10 mg

DOSE Reconstitute with 1 mL bacteriostatic water. Inject 15 units twice weekly into sub-Q fat.

REJUVATIDE PEPTIDES · BPC-157 + TB-500 + GHK-CU

GLOW Blend

DOSE Reconstitute with 3 mL bacteriostatic water. Inject 15 units Monday–Friday into sub-Q fat, any time of day.

④ DIET RECOMMENDATIONS

100% eliminate all food sensitivities per your test results.

Avoid **processed foods** and **seed oils**.

Avoid gluten unless it is from organic, non-GMO flour. **If gluten / wheat is a sensitivity, it must be removed regardless of being organic.**

⑤ TOPICAL RECOMMENDATIONS

Abby Rose Skincare makes a line of eczema-friendly, oil-based herbal skin moisturizers for the face and body.

This protocol is provided for educational purposes and is intended for patients under the care of a qualified practitioner. It is not a substitute for individualized medical advice, diagnosis, or treatment. Immune-modulating peptides can trigger flares and should be introduced cautiously under professional guidance. Do not begin, stop, or adjust any supplement or peptide without consulting your provider, particularly if you are pregnant, nursing, taking medications, or managing a medical or autoimmune condition.

CLINICAL PROTOCOL · 100% NATURAL

XMA — Red, Patchy, Flaky Skin Condition

Chronic dermal inflammation from an overburdened immune system

BY **DIANA M. DRAKE, BCTN** · DMD NATURAL MEDICINE

This common skin condition is the result of an **overburdened immune system** that expresses toxins via the skin, causing a reaction at the site. Removing food sensitivities during this time is important — although they are usually not the cause, they can be a trigger.

① RECOMMENDED LABS

ATTELESS LABS

Food Sensitivity Test

Pick a food sensitivity test that fits your needs and budget at www.DMDnaturalMedicine.com.

② PHASE 1 — DETOX

RUN UNTIL THE SKIN IS 90% CLEAR

SKIN NATUROPATHICS

Derma-Detox

DOSE 3–4 capsules with meals until the skin clears. Reduce the dose if diarrhea occurs.

SKIN NATUROPATHICS

Rose Guard

DOSE 3 in the PM on an empty stomach. Run this for 2 rounds (2 bottles' worth).

To clear a fungal infection, which is likely present.

DR. DALE'S

Kidney Pro

DOSE 2 caps with every meal.

SKIN NATUROPATHICS

XMA Hista Clear (FOR ITCHING, IF PRESENT)

DOSE 2–10 capsules with meals. You can reduce the dose as the skin heals.

SKIN NATUROPATHICS

XMA Heat Clear (FOR IRRITATION & REDNESS)

DOSE 2–10 capsules with meals. You can reduce the dose as the skin heals.

③ PHASE 2 — IMMUNE & GUT SUPPORT

CONTINUE FROM PHASE 1

Kidney Pro

DOSE 2 caps with every meal.

If itching and redness return, bring back **XMA Heat Clear** and **Hista Clear** to calm the inflammation.

PROIMMUNE

ProImmune Powder

DOSE 1 scoop daily, dissolved directly in the mouth.

PURE ENCAPSULATIONS

TH-2 Supplement

DOSE 2 caps once or twice daily. Start with 2 and see how you feel.

Base the TH-1 vs TH-2 choice on your CytoDx immune-panel results, and bring it in **separately** so you can see how you feel.

SKIN NATUROPATHICS

Biome Skin

DOSE 1–2 capsules with every meal.

DR. DALE'S

Digest Pro

DOSE 2 capsules in the AM & PM, and before every meal.

REJUVATIDE PEPTIDES · IMMUNE MODULATOR

Thymosin Alpha-1 — 10 mg

DOSE Reconstitute with 1 mL bacteriostatic water. Inject 15 units twice weekly into sub-Q fat.

As an immune modulator, it has the potential to cause a flare-up. Carefully bring this in and watch how the skin does.

⚠ MAY CAUSE A FLARE-UP — INTRODUCE CAREFULLY

REJUVATIDE PEPTIDES · BPC-157 + TB-500 + GHK-CU

GLOW Blend

DOSE Reconstitute with 3 mL bacteriostatic water. Inject 15 units Monday–Friday into sub-Q fat, any time of day.

④ DIET RECOMMENDATIONS

100% eliminate all food sensitivities per your test results.

Avoid **processed foods** and **seed oils**.

Avoid gluten unless it is from organic, non-GMO flour. **If gluten / wheat is a sensitivity, it must be removed regardless of being organic.**

⑤ TOPICAL RECOMMENDATIONS

Recommended clean skincare lines:

Abby Rose Skincare | Neo Genesis Skincare | Norse Organic Skincare

This protocol is provided for educational purposes and is intended for patients under the care of a qualified practitioner. It is not a substitute for individualized medical advice, diagnosis, or treatment. Immune-modulating peptides can trigger flares and should be introduced cautiously under professional guidance. Do not begin, stop, or adjust any supplement or peptide without consulting your provider, particularly if you are pregnant, nursing, taking medications, or managing a medical or autoimmune condition.

CLINICAL PROTOCOL · 100% NATURAL

Hair Loss / Thinning Hair

Peptide regrowth support, hair nutrients & adrenal balance

BY **DIANA M. DRAKE, BCTN** · DMD NATURAL MEDICINE

① RECOMMENDED PEPTIDE

REJUVATIDE · INJECT + TOPICAL

REJUVATIDE PEPTIDES · USE BOTH WAYS

GHK-Cu

INJECT Reconstitute to the top of the bottle neck with bacteriostatic water. Inject 8 units into sub-Q fat, 5 days per week.

TOPICAL APPLICATION

Apply several drops of the peptide directly to the scalp and the areas of hair loss. It can be applied straight, or diluted with a **100% Hyaluronic Acid serum** to make a topical treatment.

OPTIONAL — MICRO-NEEDLING (DERMA ROLLER)

If able, apply the serum and then use a "derma roller" (a small handheld device with micro-thin needles), rolling around the balding areas of the scalp. The micro-needling helps drive the peptide in, but is like a skin treatment — there may be some downtime and sensitivity. You may repeat once weekly, or as the skin allows.

⚠ **Do not use on broken skin.** If irritation occurs, do not re-do it until the sensitivity has gone down.

② SUPPLEMENTS

DR. DALE'S

Hair Stim Homeopathic

DOSE 2 sprays above the tongue, AM & PM. 5 days on, 2 days off.

NEW CHAPTER

Hair, Skin & Nail Supplement

DOSE Daily.

DR. DALE'S · ADRENAL SUPPORT

Optimal Multi-Pro

DOSE 2 caps with breakfast.

DR. DALE'S · ADRENAL SUPPORT

Adaptogen Pro

> **DOSE** 2 caps with lunch.

③ DIETARY RECOMMENDATIONS

Remove caffeine. Caffeine affects the adrenals negatively and interferes with homeopathic remedies.

This protocol is provided for educational purposes and is intended for patients under the care of a qualified practitioner. It is not a substitute for individualized medical advice, diagnosis, or treatment. Micro-needling should only be done on intact skin with a clean device; stop if irritation develops. Sudden or patchy hair loss can have underlying causes worth evaluating. Do not begin, stop, or adjust any peptide or supplement without consulting your provider, particularly if you are pregnant, nursing, taking medications, or managing a medical condition.

CLINICAL PROTOCOL · 100% NATURAL

Overly Rosy Facial Complexion

Facial redness rooted in the stomach & small intestine

BY **DIANA M. DRAKE, BCTN** · DMD NATURAL MEDICINE

This condition is often a reflection of an **immune issue in the stomach and small intestines**.

① RECOMMENDED LABS

Food Sensitivity Testing

QUEST DIAGNOSTICS

H. Pylori Breath Test

Is Phase 1 needed? If H. Pylori is confirmed, follow Phase 1 (removal of the infection). If H. Pylori is **not** present, skip Phase 1. — **The diet must be followed for the entire protocol** and is very important.

② PHASE 1 — H. PYLORI REMOVAL

6–8 WEEKS · ONLY IF CONFIRMED

Mastic Gum

DOSE 500 mg twice daily, between meals.

DR. DALE'S

Berberine Pro

DOSE 1 capsule with meals.

Deglycyrrhizinated Licorice (DGL)

DOSE 380 mg chewable, 15–20 minutes before meals.

⚠ DO NOT TAKE IF YOU HAVE HIGH BLOOD PRESSURE

Zinc Carnosine

DOSE 75 mg twice daily with meals.

MICROBIOME LABS

Pylo Guard

DOSE 1 capsule daily.

ONGOING SUPPORT — MAST CELL & HISTAMINE

CONTINUE THROUGH ALL PHASES

DR. DALE'S

Systemic Enzyme Pro

DOSE 1–2 caps twice daily, between meals.

SKIN NATUROPATHICS

XMA Hista-Clear

DOSE 2 capsules with each meal.

③ PHASE 2 — REPAIR LINING & REPOPULATE STOMACH ACID

6–8 WEEKS

You may stay on the ongoing mast-cell / histamine support during this phase as well.

L-Glutamine

DOSE 3,000–5,000 mg per day.

Aloe Vera Inner Fillet

DOSE 2–4 ounces daily, between meals.

Marshmallow Root Tea

DOSE Drink throughout the day.

REJUVATIDE PEPTIDES · IMMUNE SUPPORT

Thymosin Alpha-1

DOSE Reconstitute with 2 mL bacteriostatic water. Inject into fatty tissue (stomach, back of arm, top of buttocks, or thigh), AM or PM.

ACUTE (< 2 YEARS): 20 units, 1×/day, 5 days in a row.

CHRONIC (> 2 YEARS): 15 units, 2 doses per week, 8 weeks on, 8 weeks off.

Stomach Acid Re-population — HCl

Rebuild stomach acid with Betaine HCl. See the **Stomach Acid Rebuilding** protocol for the full titration method.

④ PHASE 3 — MICROBIOME REPOPULATE & REBALANCE

Stop Phase 2, and continue the ongoing mast-cell / histamine support.

SKIN NATUROPATHIC

Biome Skin

DOSE 1 capsule with each meal.

PROIMMUNE

ProImmune Powder

DOSE 1 scoop daily, dissolved directly in the mouth.

⑤ DIET — NONNEGOTIABLE

- **✗ Coffee**
- **✗ Sugar (soda, candy, sweets, baked goods, granola, honey, agave)**
- **✗ Spicy foods**
- **✗ Alcohol**
- **✗ Energy drinks**
- **✗ Fermented foods (kombucha, yogurt, kefir, kimchi, sauerkraut)**

This protocol is provided for educational purposes and is intended for patients under the care of a qualified practitioner. It is not a substitute for individualized medical advice, diagnosis, or treatment. Do not take DGL if you have high blood pressure. HCl titration is not appropriate with an active ulcer. Do not begin, stop, or adjust any supplement or peptide without consulting your provider, particularly if you are pregnant, nursing, taking medications, or managing a medical condition.

Chapter 9:
Sleep Health

Sleep is such an important part of your health and so many things affect it. From the mattress you sleep on, the light your intake, to proper neurotransmitter production in your gut. Finding the root cause of your sleep issues is important because you may notice that what works on one person doesn't work on another when it comes to taking a sleep supplement. In my practice I have found the following causes to interfere with healthy sleep, you may have one or more of these issues if you are not sleeping well.

- Improper neurotransmitter production - did you know that neurotransmitters are mostly made in your gut? That means, healthy gut = healthy sleep
- Stress / busy brain
- Food sensitivities consumed at dinner
- Over-exposure to EMF's - causing issues with pineal gland secretions - particularly melatonin) and overall circadian rhythm dysfunction.
- Over exposure to blue light in the evening - causing issues with pineal gland secretions (particularly melatonin)
- High cortisol in the evening caused by adrenal imbalance
- Caffeine consumption daily - even if only before 3pm

Although low melatonin may be an issue for you, I do not recommend taking melatonin as it will cause the atrophy of your pineal gland. Atrophy of a gland is when it stops secreting because it has become reliant on something you have taken. Instead, it is better to understand the imbalances so that the body can correct these issues and native production is restored. As far as your mattress is concerned, most mattresses are made with toxic materials and sprayed with fire retardant chemicals. If you do not already have a natural mattress, I highly recommend getting into one when it's time to replace your current mattress. Before trying a bunch of supplements to see if they work for you, I recommend a highly targeted approach of testing your neurotransmitters, food sensitivities and hormones. This will give you all the data you need to make an informed decision about a precise supplemental protocol for you. Because I am not an expert on neurotransmitters, I always run the labs through AI and ask the chat bot about sleep. I recommend this for anyone who wants a clear picture of what is going on and where to go from there. The following protocol has very general recommendations for sleep - but this protocol will need to be enhanced and customized to you per your lab results. This will take working with AI or a practitioner to get you the correct protocol.

CLINICAL PROTOCOL · 100% NATURAL

Sleep Balancing

Neurotransmitter, circadian & adrenal support for healthy sleep

BY **DIANA M. DRAKE, BCTN** · DMD NATURAL MEDICINE

① RECOMMENDED TESTING

ZRT LABORATORY

Neurotransmitter Test

Tells you what is low and high.

ACCESS MEDICAL LABS

Salivary Adrenal Panel

For melatonin and cortisol levels.

ALLETESS LABS

Food Sensitivity Testing

All of these are available at the DMD Natural Medicine "Lab Shop."

② LIFESTYLE FOR HEALTHY SLEEP

1. **Get full-spectrum daylight in your eyes** with no glass in between (no windows or glasses). See the morning, noon, afternoon, and twilight light — ideally about 10 minutes of each per day.
2. **Remove food sensitivities** at dinner meals.
3. **Stop watching TV at night** and stay off your phone and computer. Read, do yoga, or meditate instead.
4. **Aim for one elimination per meal eaten the day before** (3 meals = 3 eliminations). If you're not, work on gut health — a good place to start is Dr. Dale's Microbiome Terrain Pro and Digest Pro.
5. **If you wake to urinate,** restrict water and liquids to nothing after 7 PM.
6. **If you drink caffeine,** stop by weaning off slowly over a 30-day period to give your body and adrenals time to adjust.
7. **If you use melatonin to sleep,** wean off slowly and instead take the precursors to melatonin — **5-HTP** and **L-Tryptophan** (yes, take both).

③ RECOMMENDED PEPTIDES

REJUVATIDE PEPTIDES

REJUVATIDE PEPTIDES · DELTA SLEEP INDUCING PEPTIDE

DSIP

> DOSE Reconstitute with 1 mL bacteriostatic water. Take 5–40 units before bed, increasing by 5 units per night until you find your dose response (over about 4 weeks), then rest for a couple of weeks.

This will only help if your body cannot get into **Delta** sleep on its own. If it doesn't help, this is not the right fix for your issue — it points to upstream neurotransmitter production that needs to be corrected. You'll know within a couple of weeks.

⚠ IF AT ANY POINT WHILE TITRATING UP YOU SLEEP WORSE THAN USUAL, STOP IMMEDIATELY

INJECTABLE COENZYME · RESTORES CIRCADIAN RHYTHM

NAD+ — 500 mg

> DOSE Reconstitute to the top of the bottle neck with bacteriostatic water. Begin higher at 100–200 units twice weekly on the same day for 2 weeks, then reduce to 100 or 50 units as a maintenance dose. Inject into sub-Q fat.

④ SUPPLEMENTS

DR. DALE'S

Neurobalance Pro Homeopathic Spray

> DOSE 1–4 oral sprays before bed.

DR. DALE'S · ADRENAL BALANCE

Adaptogen Pro

> DOSE 2–4 caps before bed.

MICROBIOME LABS

Zen Biome Sleep

> DOSE As directed, before bed.

Neurotransmitter-Targeted Support per your labs

> PER LABS Depending on your neurotransmitter results, you may also need **GABA**, **SAM-e**, specific individual **amino acids**, and/or **L-Tryptophan**.

Not sure which to use? Drag your lab results into an AI assistant and ask which combination from this list will best balance your results — then bring each one in one at a time.

⑤ NERVINE & RELAXING HERBS

CALM THE NERVOUS SYSTEM FOR SLEEP

Calming nervine herbs to support sleep. Use as teas, tinctures, or capsules — alone or in a blend — and bring them in **one at a time** so you can see how each one affects you:

Valerian root — sedative; eases sleep onset. · **Passionflower** — quiets a racing mind. · **Lemon balm** — gently relaxing and mood-soothing. · **Chamomile** — a soft bedtime tea. · **California poppy** — supports staying asleep. · **Skullcap** — calms an overactive nervous system. · **Magnolia bark** — helps lower evening cortisol.

This protocol is provided for educational purposes and is intended for patients under the care of a qualified practitioner. It is not a substitute for individualized medical advice, diagnosis, or treatment. Do not look directly at the sun; get daylight exposure safely. Persistent insomnia, loud snoring, or gasping in sleep should be evaluated for underlying conditions such as sleep apnea. Do not begin, stop, or adjust any peptide or supplement without consulting your provider, particularly if you are pregnant, nursing, taking medications (including sleep or psychiatric medications), or managing a medical condition.

CLINICAL PROTOCOL · 100% NATURAL

Interrupted Breathing While Sleeping

Supporting healthy oxygenation during sleep

BY **DIANA M. DRAKE, BCTN** · DMD NATURAL MEDICINE

While there are no supplements that can change your breathing pattern during sleep, what matters is getting **oxygen to the heart** while your intake is reduced. This protocol is centered on healthy oxygenation, so the body can best utilize the oxygen it does get while you sleep.

⚠ **Get properly evaluated.**
Interrupted breathing during sleep (sleep apnea) is a medical condition. This protocol supports oxygenation but does **not** replace a proper evaluation — such as a sleep study — or prescribed treatment. Please have it assessed by your provider.

① OXYGENATION SUPPORT

DR. DALE'S

Oxygen Pro

DOSE 20 drops in well-mineralized water (electrolytes & minerals added), 3 times daily — AM, afternoon & PM.

Using **sea salt** in your water is recommended for best conductivity.

PURE ENCAPSULATIONS

Hawthorn Extract

DOSE 1 capsule 3×/daily, between meals.

② NITRIC OXIDE SUPPORT

RE-SYNC RECOVERY

Nitric Oxide Blend

DOSE 1 scoop daily.

Nitric oxide (NO) is a gas produced in the body from dietary nitrates and amino acids that helps regulate blood flow and other vital functions.

LOW NITRIC OXIDE IS LINKED TO

Heart disease · Arterial plaque formation · Coronary artery disease · Erectile dysfunction · Poor circulation · Diabetes · Alzheimer's · Autoimmune & inflammatory conditions · Mitochondrial & age-related concerns

YOU ARE AT HIGHER RISK FOR LOW NO WITH A HISTORY OF

Long-term antacid drugs (Rx & OTC) · Alcohol-based commercial mouthwash · Over-sterile oral hygiene · Chronic ibuprofen use · Overuse of antibiotics · High sugar & carb diets · Lack of exercise · Toxic overburden (smoking, air pollution, heavy metals)

Taking a nitric oxide support product is a good idea as you age, especially if you have or are concerned about the issues above. You can test your levels using oral **nitric oxide test strips**.

③ IF YOU ARE OVERWEIGHT — GLP-1 PEPTIDE

REJUVATIDE PEPTIDES · SINGLE AGONIST

Metabolic Peptide (GLP-1)

DOSE Reconstitute with 1 mL bacteriostatic water. Inject once weekly on the same day — begin at 5 units and titrate up toward 25 units until you find your dose response. Cycle 12 weeks on, 4 weeks off.

Studies now show that sleep apnea related to obesity can be improved by a GLP-1 agonist peptide. Your dose response will feel like the "food chatter" in your brain lessening, so you can make better food decisions. **Do not over-use to the point of no hunger and rapid weight loss.**

This protocol is provided for educational purposes and is intended for patients under the care of a qualified practitioner. It is not a substitute for individualized medical advice, diagnosis, or treatment. Sleep apnea can be serious and should be properly evaluated and treated; this protocol supports oxygenation but does not replace prescribed therapy such as CPAP. Hawthorn and nitric-oxide support can affect blood pressure and interact with cardiac or blood-pressure medications. Do not begin, stop, or adjust any peptide or supplement without consulting your provider, particularly if you are pregnant, nursing, taking medications, or managing a medical condition.

Chapter 10:
Mental Wellness

Chemical balance in the brain relies heavily on proper neurotransmitter production in the gut. Another important factor is hormone health. If you are taking medications for anxiety or depression, please work with an experienced practitioner that knows how to wean you off properly and understands the chemical reactions between the drugs and supplements - this is very important. Many natural supplements cause the same chemical reactions as medications, therefore this needs to be well understood and carefully monitored.

Checking neurotransmitter production is extremely valuable for both anxiousness and depressed mood. I recommend the ZRT Neurotransmitter test - this is an at home urine test kit that can be found in the lab shop at www.DMDnaturalMedicine.com . The following is a grid that can be used to determine what herbs would be beneficial based on the test results and/or the symptoms of the individual. Anxiousness can be looked at as "fear of the future", so staying in the moment and having a good therapist can be very beneficial for this. A depressed mood can be looked at as "fear of the past" that is turned inward. Working with a therapist on childhood wounds and specifically on re-parenting the inner child would be beneficial here. Anytime you are stuck on reading labs you can run them through your favorite AI. The protocols below have the base protocol listed - then use the herbal chart to customize the protocol to the exact symptoms.

Neurotransmitter	Low Levels May Cause	Helpful Supplements & Herbs
Serotonin	- Sadness, low mood - Anxiety, worry - Obsessive thoughts - Insomnia - PMS mood swings	- **5-HTP, Tryptophan** - **St. John's Wort** - **SAM-e** (use with caution in bipolar) - **Black Cohosh** (especially in hormonal mood shifts)

Dopamine	- Apathy, no motivation - Brain fog - Fatigue - Low drive/interest in life	- **L-Tyrosine**, **Mucuna (L-DOPA)** - **SAM-e** - **Rhodiola rosea** - **Gotu Kola** (gentle cognitive/mood support)
GABA	- Anxiety, tension - Racing thoughts - Restlessness - Poor sleep onset	- **GABA (direct)** - **L-theanine, Taurine** - **Magnesium (glycinate/threonate)** - **Kava Kava** (potent natural anxiolytic) - **Gotu Kola** (gentle GABAergic effect)
Norepinephrine	- Brain fog - Lack of alertness - Poor concentration - Fatigue (mental)	- **L-Tyrosine** - **SAM-e** - **Rhodiola rosea** - **Gotu Kola** (enhances cerebral blood flow)
Glutamate (excess)	- Agitation - Insomnia - Neurotoxicity - Mood cycling	- **Magnesium (calms NMDA receptor)** - **NAC (glutamate modulator)** - **Lithium orotate (low dose)** - **Gotu Kola** (neuroprotective)
Acetylcholine	- Memory issues - Poor learning - Attention problems	- **Alpha-GPC**, **CDP-Choline** - **Huperzine A** - **Gotu Kola** (used traditionally for memory and clarity)

Other considerations:
Kava Kava & Gotu Kola

- For depressed mood with anxiousness (relaxation)

Black Cohosh

- For depressed mood in females related to hormones (around period or PMS) also helps with "black cloud" depressed mood

CLINICAL PROTOCOL · 100% NATURAL

Anxiousness

The Over-Anxious Protocol — calming an overactive stress response

BY **DIANA M. DRAKE, BCTN** · DMD NATURAL MEDICINE

① LIFESTYLE RECOMMENDATIONS

1. **Remove caffeine.** Caffeine should not be used by individuals who are prone to anxiousness. If you take caffeine, wean off slowly over the next 30 days — do not stop cold turkey; it is important to go slow. Caffeine substitutes can be found at www.Teeccino.com.
2. **Daily yoga and/or meditation.** Use this tool, along with deep breathing, when you have an episode.
3. **Let it move through you.** When anxiety arises, instead of trying to push it away, tune into awareness and let it into your body. Accept it in and let your body go through it and process it — this helps you naturally let it go.

② RECOMMENDED PEPTIDES

REJUVATIDE · NASAL PREFERRED

REJUVATIDE PEPTIDES · CALMING

Selank (N-Acetyl Selank injection, or Selank nasal spray — nasal preferred)

> DOSE Use in the morning or evening. Start with just 1 spray per nasal cavity and adjust from there. Use every other day, or 5 days on / 2 days off. Cycle 2–4 weeks on, then 1–2 weeks off.

REJUVATIDE PEPTIDES · FOCUS & CLARITY

Semax Nasal Spray

> DOSE Same instructions as Selank.

Use more for cognition, brain fog, and focus.

HOW TO MAKE YOUR NASAL PEPTIDE

Blend both peptide powders (Selank and Semax) together into a glass nasal-spray bottle (a “nasal sniffer”) and reconstitute with **4 mL of sterile saline**. Use **1–3 sprays in each nostril, 5 days on / 2 days off,** or as needed.

③ SUPPLEMENTS

DR. DALE'S

Amino Acid Pro

DOSE 2 caps twice daily, between meals.

DR. DALE'S

Microbiome Terrain Pro

DOSE 1 cap with meals.

DR. DALE'S

Neurobalance Pro

DOSE 1–4 sprays in the AM & PM, or as needed.

MICROBIOME LABS

Zen Biome Cope Probiotic

BRING THINGS IN ONE AT A TIME

Also reference the herbal chart in this book for specific considerations based on your labs and symptoms. When using herbs and supplements to balance mood, bring things in **one at a time** to see how you feel. Make sure there is no negative reaction or worsening of symptoms over a **72-hour** period. If that happens, discontinue the newest thing you added.

This protocol is provided for educational purposes and is intended for patients under the care of a qualified practitioner. It is not a substitute for individualized medical advice, diagnosis, or treatment. If anxiety is severe, worsening, or accompanied by thoughts of self-harm, seek help from a qualified mental-health professional promptly. Do not begin, stop, or adjust any peptide, supplement, or medication (including anti-anxiety or psychiatric medication) without consulting your provider, particularly if you are pregnant, nursing, or managing a medical condition.

CLINICAL PROTOCOL · 100% NATURAL

Depressed Mood

Strategic, monitored support for low mood

BY **DIANA M. DRAKE, BCTN** · DMD NATURAL MEDICINE

♥ **A note on safety.**
This protocol is meant to support mood **alongside** professional mental-health care, not in place of it. If you are experiencing thoughts of harming yourself — even mild or passing — please reach out for help right away. In the US, you can call or text **988** (Suicide & Crisis Lifeline), available 24/7. Work with a qualified provider before starting or changing any of the items below.

① RECOMMENDED LABS

ACCESS MEDICAL LABS
Saliva OpenDx Hormone Test

ZRT LABORATORY
Food Sensitivity Test

US BIOTEK
Basic GI Test

If the gut needs healing, run the **Total Digestive Rejuvenation** (gut repair) protocol — gut health strongly influences mood and neurotransmitter production.

② LIFESTYLE RECOMMENDATIONS

1. **Avoid stimulating habits and substances** — including caffeine and cigarettes. If you take caffeine, wean off slowly over the next 30 days. Do not stop cold turkey; it is important to go slow. Caffeine substitutes can be found at www.Teeccino.com.

2. **Daily yoga and/or meditation.** Use this tool, along with deep breathing, when you have an episode.

③ NUTRITIONAL LITHIUM

STRATEGIC USE · NOT UNIVERSAL

Lithium in **nutritional (microdose) amounts** can be useful in specific patterns of depression — especially where there is instability, rumination, or neuroinflammation — but it should be used strategically rather than universally.

BEST USE CASES

Mood instability / cycling depression (irritability, emotional ups and downs) — helps stabilize neuronal signaling.

Depression with anxiety and rumination (overthinking, looping thoughts) — helps calm excitatory signaling.

Low stress resilience (easily overwhelmed) — supports neuroprotection and stress buffering.

Suicidal ideation (even mild / passive) — associated with a reduction in suicidal thoughts. *(Always pair with professional support — see the safety note above.)*

Neuroinflammatory or post-viral depression with brain fog — may increase BDNF and support neurogenesis.

Adjunct use — can enhance response to SSRIs, adaptogens, and peptides like Semax or Selank.

WHEN IT MAY NOT BE IDEAL

Pure low-dopamine or apathetic depression (may feel flattening), significant hypothyroidism, kidney concerns, or an already emotionally flat presentation.

> TYPICAL DOSING
>
> Microdose range 1–5 mg elemental lithium daily; common range 5–10 mg daily. Often taken in the evening for a calming effect, or split AM / PM.

④ RECOMMENDED PEPTIDES

REJUVATIDE · NASAL PREFERRED

REJUVATIDE PEPTIDES · CALMING

Selank (N-Acetyl Selank injection, or Selank nasal spray — nasal preferred)

> DOSE Use in the morning or evening. Start with just 1 spray per nasal cavity and adjust. Use every other day, or 5 days on / 2 days off. Cycle 2–4 weeks on, then 1–2 weeks off.

REJUVATIDE PEPTIDES · FOCUS & CLARITY

Semax Nasal Spray

> DOSE Same instructions as Selank.

Use more for cognition, brain fog, and focus.

HOW TO MAKE YOUR NASAL PEPTIDE

Blend both peptide powders (Selank and Semax) together into a glass nasal-spray bottle (a "nasal sniffer") and reconstitute with **4 mL of sterile saline**. Use **1–3 sprays in each nostril, 5 days on / 2 days off,** or as needed.

⚠ **Be careful using Selank with diagnosed bipolar depression or mania.** A very low dose needs to be tested first — if it causes anger or agitation, discontinue immediately. This isn't to say it cannot benefit someone in this condition; it just may not suit certain brain chemistry, so it needs to be monitored.

⑤ SUPPLEMENTS

DR. DALE'S

Amino Acid Pro

DOSE 2 caps twice daily, between meals.

DR. DALE'S

Microbiome Terrain Pro

DOSE 1 cap with meals.

DR. DALE'S

Neurobalance Pro

DOSE 1–4 sprays in the AM & PM, or as needed.

MICROBIOME LABS

Zen Biome Cope Probiotic

DOSE 1 in the AM and PM, on an empty stomach.

Magnesium Glycinate

DOSE 400 mg in the evening.

NATURE'S SUNSHINE

Mood Elevator

DOSE 1 capsule 1–3 times daily. Start at 3 daily.

Methylated B Vitamins

DOSE 1 daily with the first meal of the day.

Omega-3s

DOSE 3,000 mg total daily, divided with meals.

BRING THINGS IN ONE AT A TIME

Also reference the herbal chart in this book for specific considerations based on your labs and symptoms. When using herbs and supplements to balance mood, bring things in **one at a time** to see how you feel. Make sure there is no negative reaction or worsening of symptoms over a **72-hour** period. If that happens, discontinue the newest thing you added.

This protocol is provided for educational purposes and is intended for patients under the care of a qualified practitioner. It is not a substitute for professional mental-health care, diagnosis, or treatment. Depression can be serious; any suicidal thoughts require prompt professional help (in the US, call or text 988). Nutritional lithium, peptides, and other items here should be used only under professional supervision and require caution with bipolar disorder, thyroid or kidney conditions, and with SSRIs or other psychiatric medications. Do not begin, stop, or adjust any supplement, peptide, or medication without consulting your provider, particularly if you are pregnant, nursing, or managing a medical condition.

Chapter 11
Thyroid Balancing

Proper thyroid health begins with what I call preventative wellness. Once you have a thyroid diagnosis, it is difficult to reverse but it is possible over time. Once you get on a thyroid medication, it is almost impossible to reverse - however you can still get off the drug and transition to natural supplements to support the thyroid. Preventative wellness begins with understanding what thyroid needs for fuel.

1. Iodine
2. Selenium
3. Zinc
4. Vitamin D

Because the thyroid is a spongy gland that absorbs what are called "halogen elements" it tends to grab and store all elements within that family. Iodine is a halogen element for example but unfortunately there are a lot of other toxic halogens that you are exposed to constantly as well. And your thyroid absorbs them all. Toxic halogens kick the iodine out of the receptor site, and you become iodine deficient. Halogen elements include bromine, fluoride and chlorine just to name a few. The biggest intake of halogens is typically from tap water. If you stop drinking tap water, this is a good step but it's not enough to stop exposure because skin absorbs toxins in water as well. Therefore, a full house filtration system is also ideal. This is one of the best investments you can make for your family. At your sink, you want additional filtration and a reverse osmosis system. This truly gets everything out of the water - both the bad chemicals and the vital minerals. This is why it is important to re-mineralize your drinking water with things like sea salt or use mineral and electrolyte supplements. If you are using something flavored, make sure it is not full of sugar or chemical sweeteners.

Consuming iodized salt (table salt) is not how you want to get your iodine and needs to be avoided all together because it is not a whole food. It isn't that you don't get enough iodine in your diet, it's more that the exposure to the toxic halogens kicks out what you do have. Unfortunately, the toxic burden on Americans increases every year and women need more iodine than men because we have breast tissue. Breast tissue requires iodine to detox properly. The thyroid also gets junked up with things like glyphosate, heavy metals, plastics and even parasites. Therefore, part of thyroid health and disease prevention is proper detoxification to include metals and parasites.

The second exposure that needs to be addressed is potassium bromide. This toxic chemical is an active ingredient in fire retardant chemicals and is used on mattresses, furniture, carpet, rugs etc. It is vital that you are not sleeping on a mattress or have furniture in your home that has been sprayed with fire retardant chemicals. Bromide is also added to white flour, which I refer to as the white devil - along with sugar. White flour in America is one of the unhealthiest things we consume. It is a genetically modified blend of several kinds of wheat, it is covered in glyphosate (round up) in the harvesting process then bleached, and bromated. White flour should be avoided like the plague for good health in general, prevention of disease, and especially if you have an autoimmune thyroid condition (Hashimoto's). FYI there are plenty of places where you can buy bread, pasta and wheat products that have been made with organic, real wheat that is non-GMO, non-bleached and non-bromated.

The first thing that needs to be done in all thyroid cases is proper testing. If you have not been diagnosed with a thyroid disorder I still recommend you get this test so that you can correct any elements where you are deficient. Doctors that test you only for TSH, T3 and T4 are doing a great disservice as they are not looking at potential root causality. I recommend using the ZRT Thyroid Toxicity test that looks at:

1. TSH
2. TPO
3. T3
4. T4
5. Thyroglobulin
6. Iodine levels
7. Bromine levels
8. Selenium
9. Heavy Metals
10. Creatinine

This test helps you see the whole picture of what needs to be done to properly balance your thyroid. Please be advised that natural thyroid balancing is typically a 2-year commitment that includes proper detoxification, nutrition, gut healing and is a supplement heavy protocol. If you have been on a drug for more than 6 months you will likely need to be on an animal glandular replacement for the rest of your life.

A secondary test that is overlooked in relationship to your thyroid is a four-point saliva cortisol test that evaluates adrenal function. The adrenals have a tight relationship with the thyroid so if cortisol levels are not balanced, they will need to be addressed to support thyroid conditions. In addition to supplements, stopping caffeine, sugar and managing stress are important steps to take to support healthy adrenal function.

If you are taking thyroid drugs, weaning off your medication should be done under the supervision of your doctor - preferably the one who writes your drug prescription because it is ideal to have your doctor lower your dose as you move through the various stages of your thyroid protocol. The idea is to go down by 20% every 6 weeks, and retest TSH on the 7th week. While you are weaning off the drug it is not necessary to re-test using the entire ZRT Thyroid Toxicity Panel. During drug wean off you need to monitor primarily TSH. The goal is to bring in the thyroid glandular while the drug comes out and keep the TSH as balanced as possible. Be aware it will bounce around a little - this is why it is important to go slowly and have supervision. Ideally, your physician should be the one lowering your thyroid dosage and ordering your TSH labs as you share with him/her the plan to come off the drug. If you are working with a doctor who will not do this for you, I strongly suggest leaving them a poor review and finding a doctor who will do his/her job correctly. Your doctor is not your boss. You and your insurance company are the ones paying the doctor you choose. Always remember that you are the customer and should be provided with a service that helps you reach your goals.

Once off the drug, you may begin testing again using the ZRT Labs test to keep balancing the rest of the elements. If your test comes back Iodine deficient and bromine dominant (bromine is higher than iodine) then it is important to reverse that relationship. Remember that bromine is toxic - so when you start putting iodine back into the body and the bromine begins to excrete, this has the potential to make you feel unwell. Bromine detoxification symptoms may include:

1. Detox flu (sweating, diarrhea, nausea, flu-like symptoms)

2. Pain in the limbs

3. General feeling of unwell

If you experience bromine detoxification symptoms, please add vitamin C and magnesium to your protocol and stop taking the iodine on the weekends. This will help the body to flush the bromine safely via the kidney pathway. If you have an auto-immune response in your thyroid - meaning elevated TPO antibodies (this is known as Hashimoto's in Western medicine) Please do not start taking iodine as this can trigger an increase in auto-immune response in some individuals. Instead, it is better to take kelp supplements for auto-immune issues, this way the iodine is being delivered in a whole food version. Whether you are coming off a drug or not, TSH (and TPO if elevated) should be tested every 6 weeks.

CLINICAL PROTOCOL · 100% NATURAL

Underactive Thyroid

Detox, thyroid rebuilding & a supervised medication wean-off

BY **DIANA M. DRAKE, BCTN** · DMD NATURAL MEDICINE

① RECOMMENDED LABS

ZRT LABORATORY · URINE & BLOOD

Thyroid Toxicity Panel

ACCESS MEDICAL LABS · SALIVA

Salivary Adrenal Panel

② MEDICATION WEAN-OFF SCHEDULE

MD SUPERVISION REQUIRED

⚠ **Only wean off thyroid medication under the supervision of a medical doctor.**
Do **not** begin the drug wean-off until you have brought in the thyroid glandular.

1. **Run the protocol for 2 weeks** before weaning off any medication.
2. **Bring in Priority One Thyroid 300 Glandular** — begin with 2 capsules in the AM during the first 6 weeks.
3. **Wean the medication down by 20% every 6 weeks,** and re-test TSH on the 7th week.
4. **As the medication decreases, increase the glandular** to keep TSH balanced — find your "sweet spot." It's OK if TSH elevates slightly; keep adjusting and adding glandular capsules until you are 100% off the medication.
5. **Once off the medication,** continue to balance TSH by adjusting the glandular up and down.

FINDING YOUR DOSE & LONG-TERM MONITORING

Dose needs vary widely — some people need 10 or more glandular capsules (a high dose is fine as long as you feel well), while others need only one or two. It depends on the severity of the condition, how long you were on medication, and how atrophied the thyroid has become. With proper monitoring and testing, it is possible to be fully off thyroid medication in **7–8 months**, continuing the glandular as ongoing maintenance. Over time, as thyroid function optimizes you should be able to lower the glandular — which is why ongoing testing matters. **Test TSH every 6–9 months** for the rest of your life to properly monitor your condition.

③ DETOXIFICATION — FIRST 3–6 MONTHS

Run this phase for the first 3–6 months of the protocol. If budget-restricted, you can do just the detox portion for 90 days, then move on to the rest — but repeat the detox as often as you can while you heal the thyroid. — Remember: do not begin the drug wean-off until the thyroid glandular is in place.

DR. DALE'S

Whole Body Detox Kit

DOSE Liver Detox and Support, Kidney Pro & Whole-Body Immune Pro: 3 caps of each with each meal (2–3 times daily, depending on how many meals you eat). 5 days on, 2 days off.

DR. DALE'S

Colon Pro

DOSE 1–2 capsules with each daily meal, 7 days a week. Start with 1 and increase to 2 if you can; reduce back to 1 if diarrhea occurs.

DR. DALE'S · PARASITE DETOX

Para-Pro

DOSE 2 caps with each daily meal.

DR. DALE'S

Bio-Tox Total Metals

DOSE 5 droppers full per day.

DR. DALE'S

Bio-Film Detox

DOSE 1 capsule before or between meals, 3×/day.

DR. DALE'S

Hepatic Glutathione Pathway

DOSE 3 caps with the first meal of the day.

④ THYROID BALANCING

DR. DALE'S

BioTox Total Thyroid

DOSE 5 droppers full in the AM.

DR. DALE'S MBM/NER #11

Thyroid / Adrenal

DOSE 5 drops in the AM & PM. Monday–Friday only.

PRIORITY ONE

Thyroid 300 Capsules

DOSE Adjust the dose per your TSH levels. Take on an empty stomach in the AM, or with breakfast if it causes stomach upset.

DR. DALE'S

Nano-Ionic Selenium

DOSE 20 drops daily with water.

⑤ IODINE LOADING

DR. DALE'S

Bio-Iodine (90 DAYS)

DOSE 2 capsules in the morning with food (and 90 minutes away from any prescription medication).

DR. DALE'S · AFTER 90 DAYS, MAINTENANCE

Nano-Ionic Decolorized Iodine Drops

DOSE 1 dropperful daily in water.

IODINE MONITORING

Iodine levels should be monitored via the ZRT Labs thyroid toxicity test; levels will fluctuate. The goal is to get **iodine to the higher end of range** and **bromine to the low end of range**.

⚠ **If you have Hashimoto's, use kelp instead of iodine.**
Take whole kelp supplements in place of iodine — **Nature's Way Kelp 600 mg**, 1 daily with the first meal of the day.

⑥ BROMINE DETOX SUPPORT

IF YOU HAVE BROMINE-DETOX SYMPTOMS

Vitamin C

DOSE 4,000–6,000 mg per day in divided doses (ideally 1,000–2,000 mg per meal).

Magnesium

DOSE 400 mg of elemental magnesium per day.

Baja Gold Sea Salt

DOSE Salt your water with ½ teaspoon per day, in divided doses.

7 SUPPORTIVE

DR. DALE'S

Nano-Ionic Multi-Minerals with Silica Drops

DOSE 30 drops in water daily, for proper mineral balance.

Raw Nattokinase

DOSE 1–2 capsules twice daily between meals.

Supports healthy blood and is anti-inflammatory.

DR. DALE'S

MBM Male or Female Tincture

DOSE 5 drops in the AM & PM, 5 days on, 2 days off.

Supports overall endocrine balance.

DR. DALE'S · ADRENAL SUPPORT

Optimal Multi-Pro

DOSE 2 caps once or twice daily, with the first two meals of the day.

DR. DALE'S

Microbiome Terrain Pro

DOSE 1–2 caps with each meal of the day.

Supports proper digestion and gut permeability.

INTEGRATIVE PEPTIDES

Thyro-Pep Oral Peptides

DOSE As directed on the label.

Oral peptide support for healthy thyroid function.

This protocol is provided for educational purposes and is intended for patients under the care of a qualified practitioner. It is not a substitute for individualized medical advice, diagnosis, or treatment. **Thyroid medication must only be adjusted or discontinued under the supervision of a medical doctor with regular TSH monitoring.** If you have Hashimoto's or another autoimmune thyroid condition, use kelp rather than high-dose iodine, as iodine can aggravate autoimmune thyroiditis. Keep iodine 90 minutes apart from prescription medications. Do not begin, stop, or adjust any medication or supplement without consulting your provider, particularly if you are pregnant, nursing, or managing a medical condition.

ADJUNCT PROTOCOL · 100% NATURAL

Auto-Immune Thyroid Response

An adjunct to the Underactive Thyroid protocol — follow both together

BY **DIANA M. DRAKE, BCTN** · DMD NATURAL MEDICINE

⚠ **This is an adjunct — and no iodine.**

Follow this alongside the primary **Underactive Thyroid** protocol. **Do NOT use iodine.** Use a whole-food **kelp** supplement instead — from clean northern waters, tested for metals and contaminants (e.g., Nature's Way Kelp, 1 capsule per day).

① RECOMMENDED LABS

ZRT LABORATORY

Thyroid Toxicity Test

Looks at not only thyroid function but also iodine, selenium, heavy metals, and immune and kidney function.

DIAGNOSTIC SOLUTIONS

CytoDx

Determines whether the **TH-1** or **TH-2** arm of the immune system is dominant.

② IMMUNE MODULATION

PURE ENCAPSULATIONS · PER CYTODX

TH-1 or TH-2 Supplement

DOSE Begin at 2 caps daily, then increase over time as your TPO comes down. You may need therapeutic doses of up to 6 capsules per day.

ProImmune

DOSE 1 scoop daily, dissolved in the mouth.

Flavent Immune Drops

DOSE 30 drops in the AM & PM, under the tongue.

HOW TO CHOOSE TH-1 VS. TH-2

Take the supplement **opposite** to your dominant immune response. If CytoDx shows **TH-1 is high**, take the **TH-2** supplement — and vice versa. If you're not sure how to read the test, upload it to an AI assistant and ask which immune response is dominant and needs calming; then take the Pure Encapsulations supplement with the **opposite** name.

③ NUTRITIONAL SUPPLEMENTS

NATURE'S WAY · IODINE REPLACEMENT

Whole-Food Kelp

DOSE 1 capsule per day. Choose kelp from clean northern waters, tested for metals and contaminants.

Inositol

DOSE 600 mg twice daily.

Works synergistically with selenium on immune balance.

DR. DALE'S

Vitamin D & K

TARGET Levels should be 80 on a blood test — based on functional ranges, which are higher than standard lab recommendations.

Curcumin

DOSE 1,000 mg per day, for inflammation.

④ RECOMMENDED PEPTIDES

REJUVATIDE PEPTIDES

REJUVATIDE PEPTIDES · IMMUNE MODULATOR

Thymosin Alpha-1

DOSE Reconstitute with 1 mL bacteriostatic water. Inject 15 units twice weekly into sub-Q fat.

For immune-system modulation.

REJUVATIDE PEPTIDES · SYSTEMIC INFLAMMATION

GLOW Peptide Blend

DOSE Reconstitute with 4 mL bacteriostatic water. Inject 10 units daily into sub-Q fat. 8 weeks on, 2 weeks off.

Works on systemic inflammation.

This protocol is provided for educational purposes and is intended for patients under the care of a qualified practitioner. It is not a substitute for individualized medical advice, diagnosis, or treatment. In autoimmune thyroid conditions, **iodine can aggravate the immune attack on the thyroid** — use kelp as directed rather than iodine, and only under professional guidance. Thyroid medication must be managed by a medical doctor with TSH monitoring. Do not begin, stop, or adjust any supplement, peptide, or medication without consulting your provider, particularly if you are pregnant, nursing, or managing a medical condition.

Shopping Guide

Every product, lab, and resource from the protocols — in one place

BY **DIANA M. DRAKE, BCTN** · DMD NATURAL MEDICINE

Products from **Dr. Dale's, Rejuvatide, Skin Naturopathics,** and **Nature's Sunshine** are grouped under one store link each. All other products are linked individually below. A few practitioner-grade items are marked **"FullScript Recommendation Required."** Watch for discount codes where noted.

SHOP BY BRAND

ONE LINK EACH

Dr. Dale's Wellness

www.DrDaleWellness.com

- Adaptogen Pro
- Allercyl Airborne
- Allercyl Breathe
- Amino Acid Pro
- Berberine Pro
- Bio Age Erase (Collagen & C)
- Bio Age Reverse Drops
- Bio Film Detox
- Bio-Iodine
- Bio-Tox Environmental Detox + Glyphosate
- Bio-Tox Total Bacteria
- Bio-Tox Total Fungal
- Bio-Tox Total Metals
- Bio-Tox Total Parasite (liquid)
- Cholesterol
- Cold Guard Plus Drops
- Colon Pro
- Digest Pro
- Whole Body / Full Body Detox Kit
- Hair Stim Homeopathic
- Heavy Metal Detox
- Hepatic Glutathione Pathway
- Homeopathic Testosterone Male
- Kidney Pro
- Liver Detox and Support
- Lymphatic Detox Plus
- MBM Male Tincture
- MBM Female Tincture
- MBM/NER Female #13
- MBM/NER #1 Thyroid/Adrenal
- #2 Gallbladder MBM/NER
- MenoGel
- Mercury Detox Plus
- Microbiome Terrain Pro
- NAC Pro
- Nano-Ionic Bone Strong
- Nano-Ionic Iodine (Decolorized)
- Nano-Ionic Multi-Minerals w/ Silica
- Nano-Ionic Selenium
- Neurobalance Pro
- NuFem #1 Progesterone Spray
- NuFem #2 Estrogen Spray
- NuFem #3 Testosterone Spray
- Optimal Multi-Pro
- Oxygen Pro
- Para-Pro
- Raw Natto Kinase
- Systemic Enzyme Pro
- T3 Rescue (Homeopathic)
- Thyroid Glandular (300 mg)
- Vitamin D & K
- Whole Body Immune Pro

Rejuvatide Peptides

www.rejuvatidepeptides.com

- BPC-157
- TB-500
- GHK-Cu
- GLOW Blend
- Thymosin Alpha-1
- Kisspeptin-10
- MOTS-c
- Epithalon
- Selank / N-Acetyl Selank
- Semax
- DSIP
- PT-141
- Oxytocin
- GLP-1 Metabolic Peptide (Sema/Reta/Tirz/Maz)
- CJC-1295 + Ipamorelin
- Tesamorelin
- Sermorelin
- NAD+ (injectable)
- Glutathione (injectable)

Gonadorelin — source from **Peptide Science** (www.peptidesciences.com).

Skin Naturopathics

www.SkinNaturopathics.com

- Hormonal Breakouts
- Hormonal Breakouts Female
- Derma-Detox
- Biome Skin
- Rose Guard
- XMA Hista Clear
- XMA Heat Clear

Also available at www.DrDaleWellness.com

Nature's Sunshine

www.NaturesSunshine.com

- X-Action Reloaded (men)
- Women's X-Action Reloaded
- Cramp Bark

INDIVIDUALLY-LINKED PRODUCTS

PURE ENCAPSULATIONS

DHEA 5 mg
amzn.to/44FH14E

Pregnenolone 10 mg
amzn.to/3Rov9B2

Ubiquinol 100 mg
amzn.to/4bWFWcz

Resveratrol EXTRA
amzn.to/4yv74ZQ

L-Arginine
amzn.to/4pxxSoo

Quercetin
amzn.to/4fsdro6

Betaine HCl Pepsin
amzn.to/4vHMx1A

Acetyl-L-Carnitine 500 mg
amzn.to/4b6cXmm

Alpha-Lipoic Acid
amzn.to/4fwuKV7

Cat's Claw
amzn.to/4fmyHvr

Olive Leaf Extract
amzn.to/4wf1A3U

L-Lysine
amzn.to/4w9QBJ2

Hawthorn Extract
amzn.to/4feSjmB

Vitamin C (ascorbic acid 1,000 mg)
amzn.to/4hoO3Cj

TH-1 Supplement
amzn.to/45e7s1r

TH-2 Supplement
amzn.to/4wMbQka

MSM / Glucosamine
amzn.to/4wfcarT

Hyaluronic Acid
amzn.to/4wpBziv

Heartburn Essentials
amzn.to/3TgR1yM

LIFE EXTENSION · BIOTICS RESEARCH · OTHER ANTIOXIDANTS

CoQ10 200 mg LIFE EXTENSION
amzn.to/3RsXLsJ

Fe-Zyme BIOTICS RESEARCH
amzn.to/45bnzNk

Bio Protect Plus BIOTICS RESEARCH
amzn.to/4bUfMal

Lipoic Acid Plus BIOTICS RESEARCH
amzn.to/4wRw8bT

B-Complex (methylated) BIOTICS RESEARCH
amzn.to/4gKHF8f

CLA (Conjugated Linoleic Acid)
amzn.to/4vC26YF

QUICKSILVER SCIENTIFIC

Ultra Binder Caps
amzn.to/4whuJvx

Methylated B Complex (Lemon & Raspberry)
amzn.to/4pCJyGA

Pro Progesterone (topical)
FULLSCRIPT RECOMMENDATION REQUIRED

Pro Estriol
FULLSCRIPT RECOMMENDATION REQUIRED

Pro Estradiol
FULLSCRIPT RECOMMENDATION REQUIRED

Pro B-Estrogen
FULLSCRIPT RECOMMENDATION REQUIRED

Oral Liquid DHEA
FULLSCRIPT RECOMMENDATION REQUIRED

ADDITIONAL BRANDS

Nordic Naturals Algae Omega
amzn.to/4wfe63D

Nature's Way Kelp 600 mg
amzn.to/4wmkTIU

New Chapter Hair, Skin & Nail
amzn.to/4wZdajU

My Kind Organics Whole Food Vitamin C
amzn.to/3Tcb0yG

Designs for Health Quercetin & Nettles
amzn.to/4gUsfOV

Microbiome Labs Pylo Guard
amzn.to/4wZdGOS

Microbiome Labs Zen Biome Cope
amzn.to/4b6VsSZ

Pendulum GLP-1 Probiotic Pro
amzn.to/4puMVPL

Vital Nutrients Ultra-Pure Fish Oil 700
amzn.to/4wkzgxa

Monolaurin (Ecological Formulas)
amzn.to/4wZYTmZ

Re-Sync Recovery Nitric Oxide Blend
resyncproducts.com code DRDRAKE — 10% off

Natura Health Meno-Breeze
amzn.to/4gJF7qV

Natural Factors Chewable Ginger
amzn.to/4fNju84

Bezwecken Hydration Ovals
amzn.to/4fn6xjV

Thorne Vitamin D (10,000 IU)
amzn.to/44BXxCN

Integrative Therapeutics Tri-Magnesium (2-pack)
amzn.to/4ywxmuX

Douglas Labs Zinc Picolinate
amzn.to/4pxHfEA

EPIC-T
amzn.to/3RNvFbV

ProImmune
amzn.to/4fs9kbJ

Flavent Immune Drops
FlaventRelief.com code DRAKE10 — 10% off

TOPICAL SKINCARE & COMFREY

Sven's Island Topical Care ECZEMA & SKIN
amzn.to/3TcrcQp

NeoGenesis
artofskincare.com

Norse Organics
amzn.to/4fczlgi

Christopher's Original Comfrey Ointment
amzn.to/3T2fGXX

Christopher's Complete Tissue & Bone Ointment
amzn.to/4wZh9No

ANY QUALITY BRAND

CHOOSE A TRUSTED SOURCE

These are widely available — choose a clean, reputable brand:

Mastic Gum · DGL (Deglycyrrhizinated Licorice) · Zinc Carnosine · L-Glutamine · Aloe Vera Inner Fillet · Marshmallow Root Tea · Inositol · Curcumin · Magnesium Glycinate · Magnesium Oxide · Methylated B Vitamins · Omega-3s · Vitamin C · Zinc · Oregon Grape Capsules · 5-HTP · L-Tryptophan · Nutritional Lithium · Colloidal Silver · 100% Hyaluronic Acid Serum · Turmeric · Boswellia · Ginger · Willow Bark · Comfrey (dried leaf/root) · Celtic Sea Salt

Equipment & at-home therapy:

Bacteriostatic water · Neti pot · Derma roller · Nitric oxide test strips · Hydrogen peroxide · Epsom salts · Coconut oil · Sea moss gel

DIET & COFFEE SWAPS

Teeccino (coffee alternative)
Teeccino.com

DandyBlend (dandelion coffee)
DandyBlend.com

The Fermenting Fairy (kombucha)
TheFermentingFairy.com

Vandy Crisps (beef-tallow chips)
vandycrisps.com

ORDERING LABS

Order all lab tests through → www.DMDNaturalMedicine.com ("Order Labs")

Easy-to-order blood serum labs → www.UltaLabTests.com

ZRT — Cardiometabolic · ZRT — Thyroid Toxicity · ZRT — Neurotransmitter · ZRT — 4× Cortisol · Access Medical — OpenDx Saliva Hormone Supreme · Access Medical — Saliva Hormone w/ 4× Cortisol · Quest — H. Pylori Breath · Doctor's Data — 3-Day Parasitology · Mosaic — Glyphosate Urine · Mosaic — MycoTOX · Quicksilver — Metals Combo / Total Metals · Diagnostic Solutions — CytoDx · TruDiagnostic — TruAge · US BioTek — GI-Basic Profile · Ulta Lab Tests — LH & FSH · York Test — Food Sensitivity · Methylation Genomics · Telomere Length · OAT (Organic Acid Test) · Iron / B12 / Copper · A1C & Glucose

RESOURCES

PRESCRIPTION PEPTIDES & HORMONE REPLACEMENT THERAPY

Requires a virtual session with an MD.

www.DMDnaturalMedicine.com — "Peptides & HRT"

DIANA'S PRIVATE PRACTICE — 1:1 APPOINTMENTS

A premium option including private meetings, personalized protocols, and follow-ups, with direct coaching and access for the duration of your protocol.

www.DMDnaturalMedicine.com

SKOOL PLATFORM & ONLINE COMMUNITY

Free resources and master classes to run the protocols with a deeper understanding of your labs and root causes. $49/month includes monthly open group Q&A sessions.

skool.com/dmd-natural-medicine

FOLLOW ALONG

TIKTOK Diana M Drake YOUTUBE Diana M Drake Natural Medicine

INSTAGRAM DMD Natural Medicine · DrDaleWellness LINKEDIN Diana M Drake

Product links are provided for your convenience and may include affiliate links. Discount codes are noted where available. Practitioner-grade items marked "FullScript Recommendation Required" are dispensed through a professional account. This guide accompanies the protocols and is for educational purposes only; it is not medical advice. Always work with your qualified provider before beginning any supplement, peptide, hormone, or lab protocol.

www.ingramcontent.com/pod-product-compliance
Lightning Source LLC
LaVergne TN
LVHW062040101126
852251LV00026B/341